Red

Pill

An Awakened Man's Guide to Money

(Alpha Male Strategies to Avoid Female Manipulation)

Joshua Dalton

Published By **Ryan Princeton**

Joshua Dalton

*Red Pill: An Awakened Man's Guide to Money
(Alpha Male Strategies to Avoid Female
Manipulation)*

ISBN   978-1-7774561-2-2

No part of this guidebook shall be reproduced in any form without permission in writing from the publisher except in the case of brief quotations embodied in critical articles or reviews.

Legal & Disclaimer

Table Of Contents

Chapter 1: Find Your Values 1

Chapter 2: What Is The Definition Of
Conviction? 12

Chapter 3: What Sort Of Lifestyle Will I
Live? 20

Chapter 4: Why Is This Happening? 31

Chapter 5: Do You Recognize Yourself? . 41

Chapter 6: The Efficiency Lifestyle 50

Chapter 7: Story 62

Chapter 8: Why Do My Eyes Hurt? 66

Chapter 9: The Secret 68

Chapter 10: Wake Up 73

Chapter 11: Welcome To The Matrix 78

Chapter 12: Alter The Settings Of Your
Mind 85

Chapter 13: Agents To Allies 95

Chapter 14: The Secret To Success 105

Chapter 15: The Method 113

Chapter 16: Eternal Health.................... 115

Chapter 17: The Secret To Eating Healthy
.... 127

Chapter 18: Why Theory? 135

Chapter 19: Why Descriptive?............. 141

Chapter 20: Demand And Supply 150

Chapter 21: The Pitcairn Experiment ... 161

Chapter 1: Find Your Values

Many men live their lives without having the values they hold dear. Actually, the majority of men live their lives only with just one value. Women. The majority of men are raised by one mother, or sometimes each parent, in a very mother-dominated home in which the mother is the one who teaches that her son to love women due to the kind of treatment she would've liked to have received when she was at her best. Men may grow up with mother abusers who used all their frustration and anger that was meant for fathers to wreak havoc on their children because they looks like his dad'. Men may grow up with parents who were absent and didn't have anything about their children. Certain men were raised by mothers who were first women and mothers last but never took their father's side, or backed his position on any issue. No matter what the situation, men generally end up being sexy to some degree or other and with a only a few occasions.

This can cause different results for men. Some become familiar with the term "red pill" at an early age, but don't know of the term, whereas others are blue pill-bound and believe that more sexiness and kindness towards women and society can earn the love of their loved ones and kindness. Men who are exposed to how ridiculous the world has become are usually considered villains since they decide to prioritize themselves and then taint the rest of society. Men who continue to be a part of the system are seen as "real" men since everyone else gets benefit from them and not just the men. The gynocentric culture of women receiving what they want when they'd like, without consequence has caused more harm and destruction to men than fear of failing or limiting views, as well as conflict ever be combined. Men who make a conscious decision and begin to look out to be number one usually have more favorable circumstances. . . But it's not much better.

The blue pillman and the red pill conscious man share a commonality similar to the way that a heroes and villains in every film do. . . Both are operating under the same paradigm which is favorable to social justice, which is female empowerment to the at the expense of men. Consider it for one second.

We'll review of the Bad Boys interaction. . .

Boy develops into an amiable guy who is unflinching and obedient to women in line with what the society agenda is. After being disqualified by women and experiencing little success with sexual relationships or falling into a romance with a woman who takes his heart out of his chest before crashing into the floor He's devastated emotionally and chooses to get off every female's body from now on, to become the unpopular guy.

The thing that most people aren't aware of about this is the fact the fact that it's embedded into gender-based society, making males and females alike to themselves, bringing them closer with their basic instincts, and removing them further from the higher levels of their brains making them easier to manage.

How? Thank you for asking!

The Nice Guy and the Bad Boy are both the same person. They both grew up in with the same values, hold the same beliefs, share similar beliefs regarding limits as well as being influenced with the same gender-centric programming and eventually desire identical things. Only difference is that some get married, while some don't. It is striking the fact that both of them define their existence solely on the basis of the success they have with women.

A Nice Guys licks his wound and searches for an appropriate master and his Bad Boy becomes petty and angry, much like his mother. He chooses to take women's genitals and throw them off to the side in order to get a better deal from the hurt. However, the problem is that regardless of how many fucks the guy gets, regardless of how many cheeks he is clapping regardless of how hard it is that he has his dick pulled it still feels empty within.

Both men contribute to the agenda of gynocentricity. They are both gynocentric. Bad Boy is placed on the pedestal of women who, for the most part, are snarky, while they are a lot more sexy than the Nice Guy is placed on an equally high pedestal and is given the status as a'real' man instead of'real simp'. The good guy is seen as every young, sexually enthralled woman's dream man, and the idea is that if one could just create him to look than a nice man to their eyes, then everything will look perfect, but they don't realize the reason why they do not like the man in the first place. The older women that are beyond their peak need to be served by younger, sexually competent females need adventure, thrills, and a rollercoaster of emotions, and a nice man does not exactly meet the needs of the girls.

So, what exactly does matter to understanding your beliefs?

Once again, thank you so much for having have asked!

Understanding your values is being aware that you're free from anything. Understanding your values is understanding the type of life you would like to lead, what kind of relationship desire to develop with your partner. Which kind of people do are you with, and what sort of delusion to stay clear of Knowing the person you are and the kind of persona you have as well as observing all the debauchery, degeneracy and disgrace that is going on in front of you and choosing not to be part of the same. This means operating and living in an exact way to eliminate the nonsense from your existence to be at peace and live your peace and harmony.

However, that does not mean that you will not experience the ups and downs, nor does it mean the fact that you will not have to face some of the nonsense. Everyone does. That's life. But, you can reduce the amount of crap through defining your priorities and having clear limits on the kind of things you'll or will never accept in your own life. Set the bar for others and yourself you and putting your priorities and goals in order, you can start to create the right set of circumstances which puts you in the vicinity to a higher category of women as well as a more prestigious group of individuals, and a greater quality of life.

What are the values of today?

The questions keep popping up. great questions, don't?

Here are my personal values: Honor, Respect Honesty, Integrity, Family and Love.

In lieu of going into the details of the meaning of these values (I currently have a guidebook for these values) Instead, I'll explain the value these values bring to me. They give me an idea of where I am going and help me envision what kind of person I would like to be. One who places his self-esteem first, who honours the commitments he makes, acts with a high degree of integrity, recognizes the value of functioning and healthy family structures and recognizes that true love exists and is able to discern between it and mindless love.

Values are a guideline for forming your character. They provide you with a outline of your life. Values are the thing that is that you are able to determine what they represent and you do not have to believe that my values are the only ones I have, they're only an example. They are part of a larger framework of values, which is an assortment of values adhere to always. When you are aware of your values, then you are aware of which actions are in line with them and are able to discern the nonsense coming out of the distance. Values allow you to step away, make yourself accountable and other people accountable and to take the appropriate actions whenever someone is trying to bully you or you, and not to accept being considered a lesser human being.

It is what it means having values, and it's important to understand which values they represent. If you realize that you're not following your own inaccurate values. It is possible to change them. When you realize that the whole way of thinking of how you view life is incorrect. Change your perspective. When you discover the truth, everything you thought you understood about women and feminine nature is not true. Change it. When you realize that the only thing you truly need is a relationship that lasts for a long time with a particular woman, it's unlikely that she's going to be charming and undermine the entire thing since she's accustomed to turmoil. Change it.

In the end, you must know your ideals and be aware of what you're looking for in a life. Also, you will be able to manage your time and gradually, but surely, grow into the masculine and strong man you'd like to become. The pursuit of values is an individual one and you are the only one who can determine the kind of values you'll want. Whatever you decide ensure that they align with you and you can apply them to your personal way of life.

Good luck finding your strengths.

Conviction

For those who have been following me for a long time are aware of my speak about the importance of conviction and ways to develop it within yourself. The advantages of conviction are greater than confidence, and what's the difference between them. We'll get deep into the conviction power of your beliefs as well as the reasons behind it about, and the source it comes from. However, I'll caution that it's not going to be founded on an inordinate amount of data as well as research or empirical proof We have plenty evidence of this already. But, it will be a little philosophical and spiritual. But don't worry, I'll explain the spiritual aspect of belief into practical words and provide couple of steps that you can use to cultivate the conviction within you so that you live your life the way you desire to live your life.

The preamble is now gone. . . We'll get started!

Chapter 2: What Is The Definition Of Conviction?

Conviction

1. An official statement that a person is liable for committing a crime offence, which is prompted by the decision of a jury, or an judge at an instance of law

2. An firmly held belief, or idea

3. It is the quality of proving that one is completely convinced of the things one believes in or declares

Conviction (www.eaglesflight.com)

Conviction can help overcome obstacles that is both internal and external. It is possible to face resistance in a variety of ways however having a base of conviction will allow you to remain positive in confronting it. All of these benefits of having conviction--overcoming obstacles, sparking passion, and overcoming resistance--leads to results

Conviction (www.collinsdictionary.com)

If you are able to stand up for the truth of your beliefs, you are able to believe in doing the things you think is the right thing to do, despite the fact that others may not be in agreement or agree with the decision. Developers need to be courageous to stand by their beliefs and adhere to the things they excel at.

Confidence

1. The belief or feeling that you can trust an individual or entity; confidence.

2. A state of having a feeling that something is true.

3. An inner confidence that comes out of a sense of appreciation for the abilities and strengths of oneself.

Confidence
(https://www.usf.edu/counseling-center/top-concerns)

Self-confidence refers to a belief regarding your abilities and skills. This means that you recognize your abilities and confidence and feel confident in yourself. confidence in your daily life. . . However the lack of self-confidence can cause people feel self-doubtful become passive or submissive and have a difficult time trusting other people.

Confidence (https://www.huffpost.com/entry/spiritual-self-confidence)

Spiritual Self-Confidence is the unique and tangible sense of faith that is not affected through internal or external fluctuations. You are absolutely certain. It's knowing what you even know. . . This confidence comes from the desire to be powerful and the desire to conquer.

On the surface, they appear to be alike. However, it depends on the way one is utilized and within the right context. What I'm asking you to pay particular focus on is the level of confidence they each bring. The confidence, although an important characteristic to possess can be derived from the result, logic and proof The other one, conviction isn't. The source of conviction is it's you. It is the faith that lies not just that you have an opinion, but your core of who you truly are as a human being. The belief is that you can get the desired result of becoming prosperous, be successful, and that you would be more willing to die than be defeated, and that you will not accept losing. The conviction of your beliefs overrides logic, reason and reasoning and depends more on your soul, your gut as well as your connection to the spiritual essence of the universe that is swirling around you as life force.

The confidence you have is determined by a performance, attributes and capabilities that prove to your brain that you're exactly what you're claiming to be and you have actually achieved your goals.

Conviction can be found regardless of outcome. It is independent of logic, reason or the evidence that is that you are presented with by the current situation. The concept transcends being able to win or lose and has one idea. . . It will, by whatever methods necessary reach its goals.

Conviction is subjective; confidence is 100.

It's common to hear authors boasting about their confidence in their abilities, how they gained confidence of women with just three steps, using this particular steps to be 10 times more confident and are currently doing well in the world. In some instances, these claims may be true but in others, it's not the case.

What are the requirements to become a strong and well-informed man? with unshakeable integrity an individual whose core cannot be questioned and whose only thing that can be proven by faith. Complete faith, trust and even trust in your own abilities. It is not about the attributes and abilities that result from them, but what those qualities and capabilities are derived from. . you.

You are the source for everything that happens in your daily life. Your decisions. Your well-being. Your fitness levels. Your diet. Your relationship. Your financial position. Your masculinity and manliness. Your mindset. Everything is a result of yourself before you even realize that, and then look inside for the strength of your belief in yourself You lack the motivational energy needed to lead a life of purpose from the beginning. Through conviction, comes passion. through conviction, comes commitment. and with conviction comes a relentless attitude, and with conviction comes mania and obsession. Drive to succeed, hunger, thirst determination, concentration, and purpose which ultimately leads to the realization of your potential.

If you're convinced and conviction, you are aware of what you're looking for. With conviction and you are convinced, everything else is fading in the blur of. If you're convinced and you're not a anyone who gets on your side, as the unstoppable power you possess and the same amount of willpower that can allow you to enjoy video games for 12 hours without sweating and will beat any opponent. If you are adamant that you are adamant about your beliefs and cut anyone's head off who attempts to undermine them, without consideration because such recklessness in regards to your well-being is not tolerated any longer and is considered with the utmost predisposition. With conviction that death is the only option as surrender has been eliminated from the language of. There's nothing to fear or doubt and there is any uncertainty. The resilience is unlike the ones we have seen before This is similar to being the Super Saiyan God (for all my anime fans).

By relying on your conviction, you will become unstoppable.

After the motivational part is over What are the next steps that you can follow to increase the fervor of your beliefs and help you live the lifestyle you wish to live without fears?

But the truth is that there really are nothing to do. The power of man's convictions is a personal thing. There is no one collection of behaviors or actions that can ignite your inexhaustible power that is your real potential. All I can suggest to help you discover your passion is to not be focused on the money aspect, put aside your focus on yourself-improvement in the interest of being a sexy girl, quit seeking to know the female character as it isn't important and just sit down with yourself for two days. As you are sitting with yourself think about this single query. . .

Chapter 3: What Sort Of Lifestyle Will I Live?

That's it.

Then, you are able to alter your mind if you wish and it doesn't matter. It's important to ask yourself the most crucial question that you can answer and then to really think about. This introspection is to determine your answer which resonates most. When you notice a surge of vitality, your muscles of your face start to contract, you notice the intensity that you wouldn't typically experience while working out outside or exercising, you feel a shaking of your legs, a grinding the teeth, and an intensity that the majority people would interpret as the expression of anger or misguided aggression, however, it's the convictions of yours coming towards the surface. If they do reach the surface, you must identify these feelings, and then form your thoughts into a picture of your ideal. Be aware of it, smell it, feel it and taste it. Then, listen to it, swathe it in your arms by wrapping it in your whole being, and finally decide. . .

The option to truly exceptional.

Live In Reality

The Most Painful Thing In Life

You learn you were offered the lifestyle, a style that you believe inside your soul that you never destined to possess. Being raised in an environment that taught that you be a believer in the universality of destiny even though the truth is that there is no an "one-size-fits-all.

One of the most difficult things that we can experience is having to discover that the reality of life is more cold harsher, more cruel, and difficult to forgive than the teachers, parents or friends as well as the social pressures of society would make us believe. It is a nightmare to lie in bed to sleep at night and wonder if there is something wrong as you're not part of the same relationship as someone else and you don't have any family members with one of your own.

Sitting down and thinking that the way you live your life is flawed because you're different from everyone else. You think that you're deficient and ill and strange since you were never designed to be like everyone else. It wasn't your intention to spend holiday celebrations with your family to chat about everyday things such as t.v. programs, songs, what celebrities did what and with whom and watching other people be amazing as you lounge on your comfortable couch or on your bed analyzing items you'll never be able to accomplish in a million years.

It is to recognize that you're an integral part of a dark and brutal reality, which requires you to give up every dream you've ever dreamed of. to change the entire way you think about things and become something you would have decided to be in the event of a chance. Making difficult choices and sacrifice the things you've been taught in order to find what is truly what you need.

It is to let off a life which, if you consider it, gives you a brief happiness in exchange for pain and sadness because it's beyond your reach and may always remain as. It is to know inside that you are meant to excel You were designed to reach the top. You are meant to excel in your life, and you were meant to make a difference for yourself to help others by providing inspiration or as a shining model.

It is to realize that, even if you thought that life was simple that you have you have a spouse, children and a functioning family, work you do not hate, and friends who are able to hang around for longer than 5 minutes and not want to kick at them.

It's true that you'll never be able to live this way because so many people have been messed up within their heads to be aware of what it means. Even if you find a person who declares they would like it but they're unlikely commit the same effort as you perform. In fact, they'll ask that you do the entire work to make your partner and yourself content, which seems absurd.

While not everyone is living in the shadows There are some who live with a sense of the bliss of ignorance, and to them, I'm saying God thank you. This reality isn't something I want to wish to my most hated enemies. If you're living by the lies there is only one solution which will provide us with an everlasting sense of satisfaction and fulfillment. . .

To be exceptional.

The rest is beside the point. . .

The Main Reason For MGTOW/Red Pill

The realization that you've been told a lie that you can never achieve is a heartbreaking as well as a harsh reality of the. Thinking that there is there is something wrong with you since you're not living up to the ideals society has taught you to believe is even more difficult. The fact that your body and blood, your personal "family" consider yourself as a solitary and as bizarre, an unreal and flawed creature that tarnishes an honorable name for your family is worse.

A part of you which is looking to be compassionate and compassionate and form strong and long-lasting bonds. The part of you that is looking to form a bond with an extended family, to have children, and create an abundance of a family. It is also realizing that some of you was never really there.

You are being conditioned to believe in an untrue paradigm that causes you to lead a lifestyle opposite to who you is, battling this false notion when you realize the reality of your situation, recognizing that you've been misled all your life, then having to break free from all of the rules and finding out why that you've always been an outcast You've always struggled with getting friends. People were at ease with you one day but then resentful the next day and girls showed them all kinds of attitudes that made you feel odd within a place that you're supposed to be into.

Each of these problems, all those things happening in your daily life, that you don't know about however you are expected to shoulder the blame for as a teenager. When you reach old enough, you're treated as men and do you know why? Men aren't worth it, they do not deserve to be treated as shite and men do evil things Men are evil males, fathers are deadbeats Men abandon their children and abuse their wives, men lie, they cheat, niggas aren't shit Fuck the patriarchy women's empowerment women's empowerment, body positivity and the #metoo movement, social justice as well as a myriad of others that make one feel shamed for the person you're born with. . . A man.

The pressure of having to face all of this for so long before you're prepared, and having to get rapidly as well as develop the mental and stoical ability to handle this kind of thing or lose the sanity you have, and possibly your entire life. It's the reality of almost all men to experience.

You're realizing that you won't have the perfect fairytale romance, realizing you'll never meet that perfect partner, realizing there's no way to ride off into the sunset. Knowing the fact that there's no possibility of a happy end and that the reality is harsh hard, cruel and unforgiving. For a man is that you're just a failure with nothing more. When you accumulate enough resources, you're an object of extracting and exploiting. It is a fact that everything is subject to condition for the environment. It is a bargaining table, and there is no remorse if you bargain without a plan.

Do you want to know the most ridiculous and reversed aspect of this?

If you eventually, with a lot of effort resolve to leave your fantasy to fully accept the reality. If you decide to follow your beliefs and begin your own hero's adventure, you're finally confident enough to stand in your own two feet and be independent enough to satisfy the needs of your own. Once you have killed that part of you that is looking for external things to admire and turn your attention to yourself and your life will improve 100 times over, you are attracting people to your life. People are looking for you to be compassionate generous, compassionate, and kind Now people are eager to build relationships with you. Suddenly everybody is impressed and would like to be with you.

If you can see this backwards-looking shit play out the front of your eyes, you realize what a cruel game the universe has played with your life and how fate has decided to play right up to your faces. Only one thing to think about. . .

Was this all about that I was looking for?

That, dear readers that is the primary motivation behind MGTOW. People being taken away from a dream and made confronted with the realities that tell you the sole option to live a satisfying life is to become exceptional and all else is irrelevant or else you'll die.

It is a fact that says people are succeeding objects, and not else.

Reality that isn't based with love but instead pressure, power struggles and unbalanced social interactions.

It's like the barren desert, and men is required to take the abyss and make it worth your time.

The reality is that you have to go to war in order to achieve peace.

The question is, what can we do about all of this? There's just one choice and that's only one. . .

Do something extraordinary, all other things do not matter. . .

Philosophy The Importance Of Philosophy

The subject of philosophy is confined to the seat in the typical library in a college, an optional course that must be taken at a minimum once if you are planning to pursue majoring in gender studies.

Chapter 4: Why Is This Happening?

It is due to the fact that the philosophy of thought has been eradicated for several hundred years. A long time of coercion, corruption power, mental games with the political and biased legislation have been enacted to ensure that philosophy as a whole is almost non-existent.

The significance of philosophy is not only for the universities and schools but also in local homes is vital for a very simple reason. . .

The philosophy of the mind provides you with knowledge, wisdom and wisdom and direction, which is essential to be moral and civilized humans and conduct your daily living in a morally responsible method.

Philosophical thinking is the way to guide people who have lost their way and the solution for those with an interest in the mind The source one may turn to discover the answers in themselves. It is a practical and practical concept to aid you to not only cope through, but also overcome any mental stress or physical situation within your daily the world.

This will be concluded with one query:

What is the reason why Stoicism taught in the universities or homes?

Strength, Stoicism, And Success

There are numerous female traits that women like on men. However, most important are power as well as stoicism and achievement.

What are these three reasons?

The word "strength" refers to the capacity to defend and obtain food items, provide shelter and meet any other kinds of physical requirements. Stoicism is the ability to utilize strength effectively and efficiently in order to get maximum results. The success of a person is the result the two previous factors, which makes the ideal man to the majority of women to get married, raise healthy children and lead a in a higher or lower quality life.

At least, this is the biological/evolutionary breakdown of it.

From a culture viewpoint, there's something more. . .

Today and age when people connect through dating websites and enjoy short hookup sessions, however true, lasting, long-lasting relationships are more difficult to establish and nurture like the story of King Arthur seeking to find his Holy Grail or Goku reaching the Ultra Instinct.

The worst part is that there's no way to change this, or even return to time back to the 1950's when things were thought to be "Golden".

But, we are able to mold our lives into the most perfect people that we can be to lead a standard of life. This is the one thing that people don't know about women. . .

They are found everywhere in ALL the life's circles.

ALL OF THEM.

In other words, no matter how well you do as a male the women will come if you can do an adequate standard. You don't need to be a millionaire or billionaire to be attractive to women. It's all you need to do is achieve perfection in your job in addition to enjoy the work you do.

The most important thing men need to know is that the desire for women's interests is not a substitute for pursuing quality and a goals. It is a waste of time and is a complete waste of your time. You meet useless and shabby people who make fun of you, abuse your and throw them off like you're nothing.

This is not an attack against women.

It's an acknowledgment that humans go through hell also. . .

There are women all over the place. The boardrooms, mansion celebrations, the bank districts as well as the fashion districts factories, and so on. Women are everywhere around the globe and are more numerous than men by at least seven times to one.

If you want to get a woman to stop acting as if it's a daunting work!

Strength, Stoicism, and The qualities that provide you with not only tranquility but also a greater quality of living. These qualities will permit you to live the lifestyle that you wish to live in your own way. They will make it hard for anyone to profit of you, and to use to achieve their small-scale goals. This will make your life worthwhile for you to live it.

The strength comes from recognizing the weaknesses you have and working to improve the areas you are weak in as you build your strengths naturally. Stoicism is the result of getting rid of unreasonable expectations and accepting that life will have it's ups and downs. It's also important to realize the most important requirement to be able to handle it all is calmness. The key to success is two factors, the first and second. It comes from your efforts, it is the reward you earn for sweat It is the goal for your work and expression of your desire.

There is a chance that you will not be attracting those women that guys and criminals do, but you'll be attracting the women who are in the area you are the best in. Keep that in mind and implement the necessary changes to your personal life. You'll thank you later.

Don't forget, this article isn't a discussion about women. . .

This is all about YOU!

The True Meaning Of Stoicism

It's time that someone from this community defined the true meaning of the stoic philosophy in particular in relation to relationship and love along with life itself. It is the general misinterpretation of what the stoic philosophy actually is and its meaning in relation to individuals has led individuals astray. It has caused individuals (and ladies) to think that stoicism simply means "suck the idea up" and "deal to it" and not taking into consideration the person's capacities and mental faculties, which is something which must be addressed if we are going develop as a species.

Then, I'll be able to explain the background on stoicism and its founding fathers However, it's not pertinent to the subject in this video. For all the philosophers who exist If you're planning to engage in any kind of philosophical thought, it is essential for you to know not just the nature of the philosophy, but also the philosophy's history since the background is crucial to understanding how philosophy operates and the way one uses the philosophy to lead a more fulfilling living.

One of my viewers requested that I make additional videos that focus on minimalism. interestingly enough, stoicism seems to be very much in sync with minimalism because it inspires people to be in harmony with the natural world. What does this refer to? Harmony with the natural world. Simply, it means to get only what you want and no else, and that's all there is to it.

We will now dive deeper into the what philosophy really implies by discussing the fundamental mechanism behind it:

The Dichotomy of Control.

The dichotomy between control and controlling was created by Epictetus when he wrote (and I'm taking his words literally) that "some matters are in the hands of us and others do not and therefore we must concentrate on only the matters that belong to us". The concept of control is one that encourages people to concentrate upon things such as our thinking of actions, thoughts, wishes as well as aversions. Everything that we are in complete control of and ignore things like opinions of other people and opinions, their office, fame, social status and other things that are outside our direct control.

The main illustration Epictetus utilizes is the tennis game. If one is stoic and seeks to keep his calm and calmness of thought it is best to think about his objectives rather than rely on an outcome or a final result. That is, he will be focused on playing to the very best of his abilities, since this goal is entirely controlled by him, not being the winner of the game (which will be a matter of limited influence over).

The Stoic philosophy doesn't intend for males to simply endure the flimsiness of everyone else's and "deal the problem" as opposed to "suck the crap up". The idea is for people to keep their calm and calmness by using the capacity to be able to distinguish between the things they are able to influence and the things they aren't be able to control, while not tying themselves to those things they are unable to be in control of.

Chapter 5: Do You Recognize Yourself?

Then, it's a good idea. It's the message I, as well as a lot of other creators have tried to convey regarding women. There is no way to influence what she does. She's bound do whatever she's compelled to do and it's your responsibility to be the same. The only thing you can do is identify when she's doing something wrong and then get out of the way.

There have been people who wrote about stoicism, and suggested seeking to make relationships be successful or to improve the performance of your job, or increase your relationships with your family and friends as well as all the good things. But, they didn't say you have to take this approach at the cost for your peace of heart and tranquility.

The Stoics tackled a variety of aspects of existence, not just intimate relations, but also many others that are similar to. They also dealt with Logic as well as Physics.

Today, the Physics has become a little outdated and logic is a concept that we can use to solve other problems, but not relationships, for an explanation.

The Stoics are also conscious about the nature of reality as well as the universe as such, they also studied metaphysics that requires higher levels of thinking above the rational scale. For this clip I'm just providing an elementary, basic understanding of philosophy, since I've just been absorbed deep into it.

What are the most important takeaways?

1. Make use of your discernment and choose the right battles

2. Know that you are entitled to the same rights and greater advantage, that women do.

3. Know that you've got just as much power and authority like she does. you have the right to make her accountable for her

conduct And if you don't agree then she's entitled to hit rocks

4. A lot of the abuse you encounter with women is due to you. Yes, it may sound like shame, but it's actually not. Don't ignore red flags. Start think with a dick, and you'll see that my words are true.

5. Being a human, you have the power to manipulate the world according at your discretion. So, whatever world you design for yourself, it's your right to create rules that cannot be changed and remove anyone who doesn't conform to those rules.

6. If you do not have a solid philosophy You'll live your life like women do wandering in a haze from one place in the same direction without a discernible direction. You'll end up getting lost all the time. This is not where you're meant to. What's the key to putting your life in order is to have the solid and sound philosophy.

Now, let's talk about the concept of minimalism. Does minimalism fit with the philosophy of stoicism? The stoics were believed to live a life which was harmonious with nature. They believed believing that cultivating virtue is the most noble thing. The result of virtue is fame, money, status and other items that are given to man. The concept of minimalism can help you determine the things you require, not the things you believe you require and reveals what you really need to be content and satisfied with your life. Therefore it is an element of stoicism because it lets to control your needs, that allow you, paradoxically to make more money and enjoy the lifestyle you'd like to live.

Actually, many aspects of minimalism's values like donating to charities and doing a good deed to help others, donating to the community through doing volunteer work, and forming an organization of like-minded members to push humanity just a little bit of the way, is in keeping with the ethos of stoicism. Stoicism is, in its essence is a way of thinking that aims to unite people and help humanity grow through all ages. Through pursuing the virtues and doing things right it is possible to not only become better people, but more human beings, and are able to lead other people in the same direction (those who wish to led).

So, if you're doing stoicism, then you're in fact also practicing minimalism. Take care of what's essential. Make the necessary decisions. Establish a structure for your day and the way that you manage your time. Aiming for virtue and the maintenance of tranquility and peace of mind is essential if you wish improve your human being.

Live The Life You Want To Live

A Sense Of Reality

Many of us living within the Manosphere or MGTOW Red Pill space frequently hear phrases like "get your life in order" or "get an existence" and "create your own universe" however, nobody has ever tried to explain the meaning behind it. . .

In this article I'll explore the philosophies behind these assertions and a little of psychology. First, let's talk about a little of existence theory.

The way nature operates is to hate a vacuum. . .across across the entire board.

It doesn't matter whether it is right or left or up, down 10 degrees left, 20 degree to right or even in the crook of a plumber's sass the nature is absolutely against vacuums!

Anything that's unfulfilled and barren needs to be filled either both internally and externally. Take a moment to think about it: when you feel that there is something missing, we will look for it (typically to the wrong areas). We attempt to make use of tangible objects from the outside to resolve internal intangible challenges.

The intangible and internal issues were caused through external factors, however our perceptions of and the ways we deal with external circumstances are an internal and personal issue that only we are able to fix individually.

We often think that something isn't right within our lives lies in the fact that we're disconnected from our soul and our perception of ourselves. If we don't feel connected to our inner being, we don't have any sense of what is real about our lives. We are just another unmindless machine acting like an automaton while life flies through, watching other people be exceptional while we're required to settle for the way we're doing, wondering whether we'll be ever satisfied and happy. Are you wondering if money, cars clothing, fashion, as well as all the material things society gives us will bring us to a complete state. . .

The answer is the definitive"NO!

47

The process of building your reality and a sense of reality is taking care of the voids in your being. Only you can determine the source of these voids, and the reasons that they are that caused them and you are the only one who can step into them and take them out. There is nothing outside you that can repair what's broken inside your own self. The money won't fix it. an affair won't make it better A happy marriage and gorgeous kids won't solve it An extensive healthy, happy family that is able to get together won't solve the problem.

Perhaps you're thinking "actually it's all I need to do is be needed to solve my problem is I'll be content. That's when I'll feel content. And then I'll feel complete."

There's no way to do it.

The void can be all-consuming. The void is one that is always taking and give. It is necessary to give something in order to receive all the things I've listed. And it is important to be the first to give it to yourself before giving the same thing to other people. Love, affection, kindness, compassion, understanding, wisdom, knowledge, respect, appreciation. You must give them yourself first before you be able to receive them from other people. If you do not give your own self these things, you won't get them from anyone else as they think you're not worthy of yourself what's the reason they should?

Morality of the tale?

Find your inner voice. Create a sense of belonging. Be Somebody. The person. An individual human being, rather than being a machine the job of a machine or an automated system. Find the voids in your life so that you're able to be able to enjoy everything you'd like and live your life the way you would like to lead.

Chapter 6: The Efficiency Lifestyle

Then, what's the definition of efficiency, you might ask? Here's what I'll reveal!

The term "efficiency" simply means that one does only the minimum necessary to survive which is to say, be able to survive. It isn't minimalist, as they distinct. It's a decision, but it's not. It means that all of the physical and mental demands are being fulfilled, however, you are able to cut out certain items that aren't important or in the least, aren't important more than others. The concept of minimalism revolves around selectiveness, picking the items you would like to be exceptional in (or just prioritize) as well as, because of happiness and satisfaction being part of your character, you can achieve your basic or enough amount that is required to be satisfied for all other things.

The key is to focus on what is important and then take care of all the rest.

The life style of efficiency in contrast is totally opposite to this. The time to adopt this style of living is in the beginning when one is just starting out trying to establish familiar with this frigid and sometimes unforgiving environment. It's fine for the duration of time however it takes between one and three years to get there. is the typical time people live the way they do. But, at the age of three, it is recommended to develop the desire, the need to change things and move to a life one of comfort. It is a problem that many get trapped within this rut of efficiency (particularly the males) and choose to stay there forever.

What is the reason that living the efficient lifestyle do good for anybody over the long term. It's simple, if you're looking for to be in a relationship, are looking to have a family, or If you are looking for long-lasting and authentic connections, living the efficiency lifestyle is one of the things that won't bring you there. Be aware that a relationship particularly one that is committed can be a significant amount of work. It requires both parties have their psychological and physical demands met, despite their diverse backgrounds and experiences.

It was a difficult via reflection and observation of what others did day by day.

Most people (and women, if they are any) would like to live an abundant social life with the people they love. Also, they want flexibility to spend their money what they like and have the opportunity to spend the bulk of their time in the company of people they are passionate about instead of working in a work environment to make ends meet.

The efficiency lifestyle can make your life less human.

What exactly do I mean by this?

This is a reference to the fact that an efficient lifestyle can be relegated to the event of an apocalypse, where all resources are scarce, and you must make it in the way you live. This lifestyle would be perfect when it comes to. But, there are so many technology making our lives simpler, especially the delivery and automation systems that allow for acquiring things just as simple as pressing keys on the keyboard (and having enough money enough to purchase it) it can be not just ineffective and harmful to your physical (unless properly trained) as well as psychological.

Okay, now this isn't about seals from the navy or war veterans or the soldiers who have been beaten to death. This is the typical individual who desires to communicate to the world and feel sure that they are there. The lifestyle of efficiency leaves you in a state that is void. If that's what you're looking for, good luck to you. If not, continue reading. . .

The lifestyle of efficiency puts the person in a state insanity, a state of invisibility, a state that is absence of color, or not being visible to the world. You might be funny and you could be quite charismatic or an individuality. However, that persona doesn't show up physically in any way, form or shape. . .you are nothing more than a lump that is able to be transformed into whatever.

This includes a puppet of an abuser.

The efficiency lifestyle is good. It's fine. If you'd like to become unnoticed, to look like a gray guy or become a social snob, then all the power to you.

But, if you're looking for an abundant social life and genuine relationships with community and a vibrant life and a lifestyle that is rooted in real life, a life that is a reflection of your character and provides you with what you want in life, eventually, you will need to give up the efficient way of life and begin the life in comfort.

The Life Of A Warrior

It is essential to adopt the mindset of a warrior in your daily living and the various endeavors. It is essential to fight to progress in your life in order to be a successful man. accomplished by a tranquil and untense test and struggle, one that is created, sculpted and forge.

Be aware that the world doesn't take into consideration your hopes and well-being in any form, way or manner. It can be interpreted either of the two options that the world isn't interested so why should you bother? Or The world isn't interested therefore why should you try to be unique?

One way is to seek validation from society and the world in order to feel accepted. The second method is to "fuck this world" and does what you want to do and then becomes the top in the field. This second option allows an individual to go into his own soul and draw out the demon that dwells in him. The monster who wants to be the best regardless of the cost.

Once you understand that you don't have to care about the world and you stop bitching or moaning about the fact that things don't work in some alternative, the more quickly you'll have the chance to create the lifestyle you'd like to lead and accomplish the tasks you really want to accomplish and leave a mark that you wish to leave in the planet before leaving.

The Spartan Mentality

The spartan attitude is the mindset of looking at everything as a problem that can be overcome. This is the mindset that is possessed by the truly exceptional (Kobe Bryant (R.I.P), Bill Gates, Michael Jordan, Steve Jobs and many others.). This is the mindset that does not worry about adversity, instead, but being excited about the challenge as an opportunity for improvement. This is the mindset that never gives up, always believing in your capabilities in getting your job done, and surpassing your expectations.

This is what we call the spartan mindset.

What can one do to create a mindset of spartan?

Another fantastic topic!

It begins with a decision. It begins when you make the decision that you'd like to alter your life in a positive direction. It begins when you are exhausted and bored of your own flimsy and ineffectiveness, as well as a inability to be accountable for your decisions and the direction they have took you in the present.

For how you can cultivate it, start with a small. If you're trying to shed weight, don't begin weight lifting 300lbs or doing 10-mile runs each day and you'll end up killing your self. Instead, you begin by removing the food that isn't healthy and then buying fresh foods. Begin by walking 30 minutes around your neighborhood each throughout the day. The first step is to read the latest articles, and maybe even a few books that discuss healthy fitness and good fitness.

It requires time. . . A great deal of time.

Let me tell you, I'm not going to tell you the truth. It can take a long time to develop this mindset even though it's only going to take you a few months establish the mindset. The lazy slob was a long time coming It didn't happen overnight and it's likely to require years to become an active star. And guess what? The process will take time.

Weight loss is only one of the many examples. . .

The key to creating this kind of mindset is the study of philosophy. Particularly, stoicism.

It may appear biased since I'm practiced stoic. However, this is since stoicism is the sole method of thought that) is a part of life and) isn't taught in schools.

Why is it that the fact that stoicism doesn't get taught in colleges matter? Since if it was the case, many students would be kicked out of the program after their first semester. It's not because the course is a disaster, but because it will assist them with their biggest challenges and show them how to become decent human beings. Additionally, money plays a role in maintaining the human situation, not the solution.

There are two major components of cultivating a spartan mindset that may appear to be counterintuitive.

Ready?

Peace of mind and tranquility.

You're probably thinking, "I know." Spartan tends to be linked to war, hardship struggles, suffering and so on. What exactly does peace of thought and peace of mind have to do with Spartan mindset?

You are a pro at asking the right questions, don't you?

OK, I'll fix the issue for you.

Peace of mind comes from an environment, and peace of mind is calm, peaceful and serene.

What is the main difference?

It is possible to physically make an area with comfort and confidence (i.e the man's cave, your home or office space.) In contrast, equanimity refers to the state of mind that can be maintained in spite of and regardless of the circumstances. (i.e. apartment gets robbed. car breaks down. losing your job and so on.)

Peace of mind is derived from the serene environment that you make for yourself to recharge so that you are ready to tackle your day with confidence.

The key to achieving peace is staying calm regardless of whatever the world or even life will throw at you. . .no regardless of the issue.

Chapter 7: Story

My story began just like many people. I was born and raised in a tiny town nobody has ever known about... with lovely neighbors, decent community, and destined for an ordinary life.

But, once I started the elementary school, everything changed. In a flash I felt cursed.

Carolyn Dweck, Stanford Ph.D. and the author of the work Mindset Carolyn Dweck, Stanford Ph.D. and author of the book Mindset, states that two kinds of mental states, growing and fixed. Growth mindsets are when the person believes that they have the potential to grow or influence their outcomes through practice or application. Fixed mindsets are when people believe they are in control over their performance and are unable to grow or improve. They believe that they're always who they are.

The people who develop the habit of thinking in a certain way were, at times, cursed. There are two methods to make a child cursed. You tell him that he's brilliant and a genius and so on. Then, you inform him you think he's stupid, dumb or developmentally disabled.

Both approaches are detrimental as it creates an unchangeable mindset that makes it impossible to change or control their life's outcomes.

As a young person I had the misfortune of being labelled intelligent. Once I was in the first and second grades I realized to my parents and teachers that I was an extremely quick learner. What would normally take the other children weeks, I would master or complete in less than one hour.

Thus, I got the brainiac, smart kid, Einstein ...

You're probably wondering, "So what?" "What's wrong?" "I would like my parents to tell me that I could be smart!"

It's fair enough.

The reason why I believe this is to be a curse is that the thoughts it generates are, " I don't have to work out I don't need to read and I don't need to do anything... The only thing I need to be able to do is show up, and things will happen for me just as they do every time. In the end, I'm an expert, aren't I? Do the work just 10 minutes prior to class starting."

It's funny to realize that this method actually worked fairly good for me up until my college days. In fact, Bill Gates said in an interview that he enjoyed laughing at students who had to study over a period of two to three weeks for the test by taking two days of study before the exam and scoring an A.

Then, in the interview Gates states that, as great as the experience was as he entered business, the same mentality and practices almost led to him being dead. From my personal experience, this has caused losing cash, time, and overall failing in every venture I've attempted to be successful in.

In the past I've played professionally-trained poker as well as engineering, screenwriting, novel writing and comic book publishing and law school. I've also tried networks marketing ...

In addition to having a vast selection of things to talk over at parties I have did not make any significant progress in either of those avenues.

When I began to fail at my latest venture, Forex Trading, I eventually decided enough was enough, and I'd take whatever steps necessary to make it work.

The secret for success became clear for me.

Are you interested in knowing about it?

Make a commitment to read the "red pill" and I'll tell you how where the rabbit hole is.

Chapter 8: Why Do My Eyes Hurt?

Although money is a major factor but there's a number of things that money won't purchase.

Can money transform your status from one of lazy people into an executor?

Do you think money will stop you from becoming a procrastinator?

Can money help you achieve healthy and good overall health?

No.

"Money just amplifies what you are already."

T. Harv Eker

If, for instance, you're someone who loves throwing kickbacks at weekends with your friends and coronas hookah, some music, maybe a bit of drinking game, perhaps a bit of FIFA...

If you have one million dollars, it's likely to not all of a suddenly be investing your funds with 10percent annual growth. Instead, you'll have a an investment plan that is set to earn 30% passive returns 30 percent savings and 40% of aggressive gains.

Most likely, you'll find yourself in Xs at Las Vegas, or the Standard in LA and at the W at Hollywood... However, rather than your home basement it's now a party in the VIP area... Instead of coronas there's a bottles... Instead of ladies having escorts, you now have promoters. Instead of an iPod, you're playing DJ songs upon the request of... The list goes you go on as well...

Chapter 9: The Secret

The key to success is directly from one of the most brilliant minds to have ever existed, Aristotle.

Student of Plato, Mentor to Alexander the Great...

Aristotle was a man of the Renaissance who's views and perspectives are the basis of the western world's thinking and thought over the past several hundreds of years.

Then, what would the mentor of the greatest winner that the entire world has ever seen have to say about his success?

"You can be what you accomplish, thus it isn't an action, but rather an practice."

Aristotle

Let's look at this from a different angle.

Your character is what you continue to perform...

Consider this. What are you doing consistently every single day?

Some people think they're always making decisions however, the majority of people live their lives by default.

The time you were up will likely be similar to the time you got up last night. If you had a seat and watched television right after you returned home last night it's likely the way you spent your day today. If you look at Facebook, Snapchat and Instagram Facebook, Snapchat, Instagram at the time you first woke up I'm guessing that's exactly what you did earlier in the day, and prior to that, and on...

We live our lives by autopilot.

It is commonplace to perform the same routines each day generally. While I am aware that there will be times that you are doing something unique, but a majority often, we typically stick to the identical routine.

I personally have took Aristotle's words one step further, and said that, yes, you're the things you do every day however, you also are the food you consume and you're the subject you are studying and you're what you believe, and you are also who you spend time with.

The type of person you're your results have in your life result from all your actions and choices you make daily.

Consider, which are my habits that are leading me to the outcomes I'd like to see?

The following item Aristotle states is

The definition of success isn't an action however, it's a routine.

A lack of action is very significant.

Aristotle refers to the mental attitude some individuals have towards achievements.

In particular, some are of the opinion that, if they earn their degree, they'll be financially secure. Also, some think having an BMW can get them the perfect partner. Others believe that helping out at a homeless shelter at Christmas time when NBC is on air is a good idea to make them feel happy.

Do you see an odd pattern?

If I take this approach and succeed, I'll have success on this subject...

WRONG.

You're sure to find plenty of examples when people who performed specific tasks didn't achieve results that they expected.

My first car was a pure white 1995 BMW 540i, complete with BBS wheels and a sunroof I'll also not be ashamed to say that the hot women weren't lined out in the parking lot, waiting for me.

According to me, Aristotle believes is that you can't succeed simply by doing something. Instead, it will be a matter of time before you achieve success.

Instead of worrying about finishing, it is better to be the scholar.

Instead of attempting to meet attractive women by purchasing cars, we should be attractive to women by being attractive males.

Instead of trying hard to make ourselves content by making a donation to a cause when it's appropriate or a good idea instead, we can become happier individuals by being a patron of a cause or charity that we are convinced of.

It is important to eliminate the notion of doing something just at least once, twice, once in a while, or whenever I can find the time is going to lead to success.

Red pill:

As per Aristotle that the best option to be successful is to become successful.

Chapter 10: Wake Up

The first step towards being free of the Matrix is gaining awareness.

Also it is important to realize that you're actually within the matrix.

Consider for a second What was the day like yesterday? The day that preceded it? What was the day prior to that?

If you're anything like the majority of people, it's likely that you don't know the breakfast you had the other day.

If you are a smart person who are out there I'm curious what you had at breakfast last night?

What is the reason we haven't remembered the events that occurred just one day? In the last few hours?

This is because the activity was routine and routine that our brains weren't bothered by recording it, or even taking note of it.

The way we live our lives is automated to the point that we can't recall the small activities we perform during the course of our day.

Why?

We always follow through with them.

Yes, I understand you have times when you consume cereal, and other times you have waffles at morning breakfast...

But, the fact is that you are in an habit of having breakfast, you are likely to do it regularly. This is a routine and routine that you aren't aware of it.

Apply this idea at breakfast time, followed by the commute to work, after which you can apply it to your routine at work routine before lunch, and finally to your happy hour. Then, you have to fight rush hour on the 91 freeway to get to home ...

I'm sure those you spoke to and the music you listened to, the location where you had lunch or the time you got to work and so on. all were similar.

It is likely that they've had the same pattern every day, too...

That is the Matrix.

Once you're conscious of the issue and have a choice of whether you'd like to become a member of the group.

The reason that awareness is vital quality is due to the fact that it takes you off of autopilot.

Consider this...

When you are aware of some thing, you start to recognize that you're performing the thing.

It is your choice to actually perform that action.

It is clear that you are in an option.

But, even though a lot of people know about things such as flossing or fitness ... they don't have the ability to make it happen.

They begin to justify their actions or defend their actions by making statements like, well, I'm sure I have to get my work done, however...

"I'm tired ... Or maybe I'm simply in a state of mind... Maybe I'm simply (insert an reason in this space)."

It is important to understand that this is not the kind of book that you read about in your head. It is a manual and workbook for how you can permanently alter your lifestyle. Therefore, I deliberately want to offend you and intend to irritate people because I am trying to get you awake.

I'm going to snap you from the Matrix with any means needed.

If you're unwilling to take on the harsh "words," how will you endure the gruelling, hard-hitting and gut-wrenching blindsiding setsbacks and blows that life can toss at you?

If you're willing to do whatever it takes to achieve your goals... Continue reading.

If not, visit the site and request a refund.

Red pill:

Change can be ignited by awareness however it isn't derived from awareness.

Do you want to know how power is generated?

Check out the article to learn more ...

Chapter 11: Welcome To The Matrix

What is the truth?

The Brain = The Matrix.

In order to change the external aspect, you need to first alter the internal.

If you want to change the outside the outside, first you need to change the inside.

You can't alter your outcomes in life unless you change your thinking process first.

Why?

As per T Harv Eker, success coach and the author of The secrets to a millionaire's mental state, "Thoughts lead to feelings which then lead to actions which lead to outcomes."

If you want to change how you think and to take the necessary action to transform your life, it is important to comprehend and be aware of the reason your brain wants to stay within the Matrix.

In "Change your routine, transform your lifestyle" written by Tom Corley, he mentions that your brain's trying to make you more resilient. That's all!

It's important to note that I didn't use the word thrive.

I said survive.

Your brain would desire to stay alive?

Based on Corley's study it is clear that the brain doesn't have any method of storing fats or glucose as energy sources similar to other muscles throughout the body. Thus, any functioning or thinking of the brain which require large amounts of energy can be taxing your body. To conserve energy and control the use of energy, the brain develops routines.

What are the habits?

Habits are automatic responses that performed without thought. It's important to emphasize the word "without thought!

Habits require little energy This is the reason why the expression "humans have a tendency to repeat themselves" isn't as cliché as it sounds.

Take a moment to think about the idea...

Have you ever thought about how difficult trying the new thing?

It's easy to start. You can keep on going for some time and then you stop.

Each time you've aimed to make a change in your lifestyle, there's always been an avalanche of obstacles to overcome. Once you begin thinking about making a change it is a constant battle with excuses, or as I prefer to refer to them as agents disguised as legitimate reasons or obstacles, problems or even impossibilities that try to keep you from.

Tom Corley's study explains precisely why we're having such difficult time altering our lifestyles.

Our brains don't need us to make changes as it requires energy which our brain does not possess a great deal of. So it's doing everything it can to keep the current status.

But, whether we know it or not, the truth is that we are either already a part of a good habit or bad ones. There is a good chance that we have either an habit of hitting the gym, or we don't go to the exercise facility. We are all creatures of routine.

"No society would like people to be wise. it's against the interests of all society. If people are intelligent that they can't be taken advantage of. If they're intelligent and are not subjugated and they are not compelled to live into a mechanical existence or to be a robot. They'll assert their own individuality. They'll have the scent of rebelliousness around their own. They would like to be free. It is the same with wisdom and it is a necessity. Both are interdependent, and nobody wants to be in freedom. The communist and the fascist system and the capitalist society the Hindu and the Mohammedan society, the Christian and the Christian wants people to make use of their intellect because once they begin to use their intellect, they're dangersome -threat for the established, risky for those ruling, risky to those who are 'haves' risky to any form of exploitation, oppression and restriction; harmful to church, dangerous to states, and potentially dangerous to countries. A wise man is alive, ablaze and ablaze. However, he is not able to trade his life in or serve others. He'd rather end his life than be slaved." The Osho

In the same way, your brain does not wish to see you change, as changing your habits will not only consume a great deal of energy, but also can lead to danger. In the end, our brains desire to stay alive which is why it wouldn't need us to expend all effort to learn new skills while we've managed perfectly with our previous practices.

When we begin anything new, take note the thoughts that come to mind such as " I'm tired and too exhausted to exercise today, I'm gonna take a break so that my muscles recuperate, and I'll need an extra day of cheating to reward myself" are just excuses (excuses) your brain making to keep you from reversing your old routine.

Red Pill:

While I'm not saying that your brain is bad, what I'm trying to say is that your brain has been operating in"survival mode. When you're on the edge of survival, and taking on a great deal of energy to maneuver and consider new situations won't aid in achieving your goals.

The brain's role isn't to help you become successful or comfortable. Its primary job is to ensure that your life a bit easier.

But, we see people making changes constantly. time do they not?

People get buff, people get rich... What happens if our minds don't enjoy changes?

Keep in mind that the brain is programmed to be a survivalist, which means it is only necessary to alter the way you think and ... to say it simply, you need to change your mental settings to go from survive to flourish.

How?

Find out more by reading ...

Chapter 12: Alter The Settings Of Your Mind

The information is extremely nuanced So, make sure you read it carefully.

Your brain does not like changes since it requires significant energy.

In order to compensate the brain's inability to make adjustments, it creates routines in order to save energy.

But, if you transform your old habits into the new one and your brain is able to aid you in keeping the routine.

There's a constant debate as the length of time it takes for a habit to take shape. I've heard it all from 21 days to 66 days and even 90 days.

Be aware that a habit is an action that occurs in a way that is not conscious and without thinking about it.

In Chapter 7 of "No Excuses,"" the success guru Brian Tracy says,

"Each action of self-control reinforces the other acts of self-control. Each act of perseverance strengthens each other action of perseverance. If you can discipline yourself to keep going, consistently you will respect and love your self more. You grow stronger and more assured. Then, eventually, you're unstoppable."

Based on my personal experience In my opinion, you'll must at a minimum, have one month to develop the habit of anew.

But, the habit will only formed after you have reached 90 days. Why? because even if you've done it for a whole month but you're still conscious about doing it and may need to keep reminding yourself to do the thing... Maybe you're thinking of going to your gym every morning, but now and then, you'll oversleep and have to remind yourself of going in the evening.

While it's nice to be at least consistently engaged in your new everyday routine, it's not possible to declare that you've established a new habit until that practice is so deeply embedded into your daily routine that you perform it daily and you don't even realize it.

My teacher Jared Martinez, aka the FXCHIEF, loves to utilize each of four different levels in the competence model.

1. Incompetence that is unconscious It's like you're not aware of the reason you're losing.

2. Concise incompetence: You recognize you have a problem, and that you require assistance.

3. Conscient competence means that you're consciously considering all the aspects you need to accomplish for success.

4. In the absence of any thought, you do every thing that allows success.

However, I can see the development of habitual behavior in this manner:

1. Month 1: Get used to your new task

2. Month 2: Become familiar with the activity.

3. Month 3: The brand new activity is normalized

Another part of creating habits is to understand that how important it is to do each day.

Again, no days off.

There are no cheat days.

It's true, I did not have the time or something else came out of the blue with bull poo poo excuses.

Be aware that agents are constantly at work trying to stop you. Don't give them a chance.

While your brain's inability to tolerate changing might seem like an issue but it's actually a positive aspect if we view things from the right angle.

How?

If you are able to remain constant with your every day activity for at minimum 1 month or so, your brain gets habitual to the activity... And since the brain isn't a fan of change this means your brain won't desire to go back to the same routine. The brain now tries to keep you from going to the previous way of doing things. Your brain will be there for you and attempt to force you into following the new routine you're developing.

Go back and read the paragraph and then again.

There are plenty of instances in the real world of this.

Ex. Rocketships use up to 80percent of their energy and fuel they consume to reach the space... When they have broken through the atmosphere the momentum of their launch takes over, and they can fly.

Ex. The most difficult part of a building is the foundation. However, when the foundation is set and the house is built, it will be completed quite quickly.

Ex. Swimming in a pool of cold, freezing water for around a minute then, as your body adjusts it, the water becomes more warm as you adjust to the heat.

Making a habit work in the same manner.

The process of laying the foundations, and making it through the initial month can be difficult but once you've done it you can make it much more straightforward.

Why?

When your brain no longer fights your brain, it ceases to hold onto the old habit, and it assists you in maintaining the new habit.

Keep in mind that your brain doesn't enjoy change... If you make a change and develop a new habit the brain will attempt to convince you to keep the new behavior and will try to prevent you from falling and returning to your old habits.

When you change your routine and change your lifestyle, Tom Corley says that our DNA is changing as we alter our routines.

Take a moment to think about this...

You don't want to drink water. However, you're an island, and only water is available ... If you sip water for two months in a row and your taste buds actually change and you will be able to appreciate the flavor of water.

Why?

Since your brain desires to encourage the new practice of drinking more water. So, it causes you to enjoy the flavor of water, which helps continue the habit.

The same effect occurs with every new habit that you develop.

If you're in the gym regularly and you're a fan of working out, you'll be happy.

If you are a salad eater every time rather than burgers you'll love salads.

It is often thought that we're unique...

Information flash: You're not all that unique!

It's not something you're looking for because you're your own You like your preferences because it's the way you're accustomed to it because that's the thing you're most comfortable with.

When a person is at ease and comfortable, it's difficult for them to make a change.

Also when someone has become accustomed to doing things their way it's extremely difficult to convince them to switch.

Red pill:

The only time when we're driven to make a change happens the moment we feel an overwhelming amount of negativity about the way we're doing, that eventually we decide to do what is necessary to feel better.

If you're really unhappy that you'll want to make a change.

A few years ago my teacher in psychology said that the whole field of psychology could be summarized by the fact that people want to get away from extreme pain and pursue extreme joy.

The goal should be to be comfortable with your surroundings which will help you succeed.

If you are able to do this then you are able to alter the settings of your mind.

If the setting in your brain change, those people who keep pushing you to the limit will serve as your subordinates and assist to achieve your goals.

Then, you was filled with thoughts (agents) which said "I'm exhausted, so let's put off work, we'll need an break." ..." When you understand the way your brain functions, you will be able to modify these thoughts. Change your thinking in order to achieve your objectives.

What new ideas can help you develop new habit?

Explore and read about...

Chapter 13: Agents To Allies

The initial step towards forming the habit of forming an habit is to create the ultimate aim.

Sure, I've heard that all self-development experts say the need to know an objective, but you need to be thinking big...

Though I'm in their opinion, I'm certainly not declaring it.

I am in agreement to Bob Proctor, the greatest educator of the mind's subconscious currently, who says all you require is something you truly would like to have. You must really desire something to the point that you'll do anything you can to achieve it.

It isn't a large-scale altruistic endeavor like saving whales or curing cancer, purchasing a home for your mother. This could mean wanting to be financially free, or buying an expensive Lamborghini and aspire to be famous.

You just have to set a goal that you truly want, and go to any lengths necessary to achieve it.

If you're still not sure your ultimate goal in life, you should stop reading and start doing it.

Here are some ideas for thought Joggers

What's something you'd like to have so badly that you're willing to sacrifice your life to get it?

What's one thing you can't live without? could be done if it wasn't for you or you wouldn't be able to do it, life would not be worthwhile ever again?

David wood, world-renown MLM coach, recounts an experience about a time when he was paid assistance on how to find recruits members of network marketing.

I've overexaggerated the tale in order to emphasize the idea...

The teacher instructed him to think that I'm with your son within my arms ... and I'm wearing a semi-automatic military matte black m-16, stuffed to the skull of his son. You were told that if you don't get just one person over three days ... That's when I'll start firing the trigger. David What kind of do you feel about being motivated to get people involved? Do you want to go to your home, watch a show perhaps check Facebook in a flash? Would you head down to the mall, the beach or even the conference center and recruit everyone within 5 miles? You wouldn't even take no breaks or take naps ... You could find someone within 3 hours or end up dying by trying.

It is what you need to reach in order to establish a new routine!

The cycle of life and death.

If you believe that this is way too much, good.

The reason to think this way is because you're battling many years of procrastination and avoiding and laziness feelings of self-doubt, times of feeling comfortable but also against your family and friends who may ridicule them or even try to get them back to their standard.

If you don't have a "life and death" mindset ... You will not be motivated enough and have the perseverance to make it through for a whole month in the process of developing an entirely new routine.

It's inevitable that you will face you will face an obstacle that is unexpected like being fired from your job, having your partner ending their relationship with you or your vehicle being towed when it happens, and your mind's agents and your negative thoughts are trying to convince you to return to old routines.

In those instances when you are able to remember your purpose, your desire that you are being held by a gun and you fail to meet it the deadline, your dreams is likely to die... I guarantee you and you'll have the drive to exercise on that day.

It may sound to be an exaggeration but it's not really, when you begin and stop, and then stop and begin ... Sometimes you do, sometimes you don't ... At times, you're in a state of mind and but sometimes, you're not sure about doing it ... There's no way to do anything.

Bill Gates, arguably the world's richest person said that from the age of 20-30, the time he was never on a time off ...

Steve Jobs was kicked out from Apple in the late 1980s, but later came back to save the company out of bankruptcy. He also paved the way for the new age of technology through Pixar, iPod, and smartphones.

Kobe Bryant, 5 time NBA champion, claims that he shoots 800 times a day.

After Adrian Peterson, the former NFL MVP injured his MCL and ACL, doctors advised him that he'd not be capable of moving his leg for about two months. Peterson instantly started moving his leg up and down slowly, while his face was swollen with discomfort. Doctor said that he had did not have anything similar before. In the following season, Peterson was awarded award for offensive player and MVP of the year award.

NFL.com stated, "Peterson rushed for 2,097 yards, a fraction of achieving Eric Dickerson's NFL single-season best. Peterson took the Vikings in the spotlight and led the team to a record of 10 wins and a spot in the playoffs. It was a season of performance, made more amazing following the reconstructive operation on Peterson's left knee."

What's the purpose?

If you are considering the possibility of death or life and your brain is ready to take whatever action is necessary to get the job completed.

The brain is a living thing, and it wants to be able to function...

Therefore, if you develop an attitude that says you're not able to live with no goal in mind the brain will assist you in achieving it.

How?

The destructive agents, the thinking that was disempowering are now transformed into positive and empowering thoughts.

"I'm tired" will change into:

They don't have to be tired.

"I'm in need of a break" is now:

I'm committing to taking off when I'm done.

The only way I'll ever be able to find time to finish it later. becomes:

We should get the routine completed quickly and then I'll take care of my shopping afterward.

One of the best things is that it means there is no need to come up with ideas like this.

The easiest way to do this is to make your own affirmations now in order in order to reinforce the new habit and belief systems you'd like.

An affirmation is an affirmation that states what you want to feel or think of yourself.

You may not be a believer in affirmations It's possible that you're doing them wrong.

Louise Hay, motivational author In an interview, Louise Hay said that many people do three positive affirmations, before deciding that they don't perform... She'll inquire about how many affirmations to help with poverty did you make? What number of disempowering and low self-esteem affirmations were you able to perform?

Do you remember how many times during the day, did you inform you:

"Nothing positive ever happens to me. I'm too stupid I'm so angry, what's wrong with me? Why am I so overweight, I'm so broke that I'm not making any savings, and girls do not seem to be able to get along with me. I'm just not the same as him. I'm just not that difficult, he's lucky. ..."

Do I need to say more?

The positive affirmations did not work ... because they were they were drowned out by negative affirmations.

If it's difficult to begin an habit of repeating affirmations that are positive to align your mind with your goals...

Make it a habit to be adamant about nothing... In any way!

If you're not able to think of anything good to say, don't say anything whatsoever... In addition If you're not able to think of something to be thinking about Imagine you have some good thoughts to reflect on.

Red pill:

When you alter your mental settings, negative thoughts that kept your down will shift to thoughts that will encourage you to stick with the new behavior.

Instead of waiting passively for good thoughts to appear to you, think of coming to the thoughts of your own... In fact, Google some affirmations that will help build the habit you're working to develop.

So, after our brain's configurations are altered and aligned in order to achieve the goal we have set for ourselves How do we make the change?

Chapter 14: The Secret To Success

"80 percent of the success rate is simply being present."

Woody Allen, an American screenwriter, director of films and actor, as well as an author

Reread the above quote slow and carefully, trying to comprehend the meaning behind it.

And then, remember the words of Aristotle stated,

"We are the things we consistently perform, so it isn't an action but rather a routine."

One of the main reason why people face difficulty time developing new routines is that they're trying to accomplish two things simultaneously.

"If you attempt to chase rabbits with two rods, there will be no rabbits."

Confucius

If people attempt to establish an effort to change their habits and stick to it, they strive in the direction of consistency and even results.

My experience is that the most important thing to be focused on is consistency.

Why?

In the end, success comes through consistent behavior.

That's why beginning and ending your diet won't result in weight loss.

If you continue to adhere to the plan every each day, eventually you'll be losing pounds.

As we attempt to begin forming our new habits, all that we need to be focused on over the next 90 days is the consistency.

My method for this is was referred to as

"just be there"

As simple as it seems. What we really want to do is be there each day.

We're still not attempting to achieve anything!

For a visual illustration to illustrate this point, picture yourself back in elementary school. All the pupils are concentrated to get an A for your class. The result. Why would they award an award to children who had excellent attendance?

Do you think that if your attendance is consistent every single day, you're much more likely to receive higher marks?

Another thing to remember is that 80% of the success comes from showing up.

Why?

You are placing yourself in a position to be successful often.

If you show up each day and showing up every day, you'll be more likely to score many more hits on base, score many more homers, get many steals, take greater fly ball ...

When you are present to work, you boost the likelihood of getting the results that you are looking for.

But, it is important to be aware that our minds be trying to hinder us from making changes at first.

In order to fool our brains into not resisting us, it's essential to make the change as easy as is possible.

One illustration I like to utilize is exercise in the fitness center.

The aim is to develop into an athlete daily, but keep in mind that in the initial 90 days, the only thing we're trying to accomplish is develop the habit of being consistent.

Some time ago, I visited GOLD'S Gym located in West Covina, and I sought out the trainer's opinion on how likely of people would be working out or even work out was if they were already in the training facility. He said that he believed that there were an 99.8 percent possibility that someone could work out when they've already been at the training facility!

Let me ask you this question: what is the probability of you working in the same place at home? In the same spot you eat in, sleep and play in? Same old, boring surroundings?

Some people may be capable of working out at home. But what's the probability that one who's lazy in their discipline, unmotivated, or a person who is prone to procrastination will be able to do the same? 30%? 20%?

Although it's possible but why would you choose to make that wager? We'll just stick with numbers.

In order to develop this new habit the first step is simply doing what we do. We must make sure that we're taking the simplest and most lazy possible thing we can come up with to start going, gain the momentum going, and finally create the habit.

The simplest and most convenient way to regularly workout is to simply go to the gym.

Take a moment to comprehend this.

In the initial thirty days that I was trying to establish a new routine of working out regularly the only thing I did was going to the gym and not try to exercise.

What is this like?

Day 1

go to the gym, then walk out.

Day 2

Walk into the gym, and congratulate somebody and then walk out

Day 3

Walk into the gym, go to the bathroom, then walk out.

Day 4

enter the gym and introduce yourself to a pretty girl, after that, walk out

Do you see the image?

We're not trying to figure it out! !

The one month that was the...

What we're trying to accomplish is make it a habit to go to the gym early each morning. Or be accustomed to hitting the gym at night after work or whatever is most comfortable for you.

The reason why this method works is that it's so subtle, that your brain doesn't make negative thoughts about it.

It's easy to use, and it's extremely difficult to create negative connotations about it.

However it is a good idea to adhere to the norms of many people do and workout the first day or God better than engage a personal trainer day one... It's likely that you'll be overworking all of your muscles and you'll feel discomfort in areas you've never experienced previously.

The shock level is not just uncomfortable however, it also triggers your brain, which is to assist you in surviving and to relay positive or negative thoughts that hinder you from undertaking the new venture.

If you've tried to be successful at something, you'll realize that failures and difficulties always arise. To deal negativity, setbacks thinking, and many years of procrastination and laziness is a lot to handle as you try to establish an entirely new routine.

The reason is that most people stop or you should take a break, cheat day, cheat week, or even cheat all year...

Red pill:

For forming the habit of forming it We should be consistent at first.

It's a waste of time and results.

Also, you won't see results until you are constant.

Chapter 15: The Method

This method works since there aren't any negative consequences to appearing. There's no expectation. There's not any muscle soreness. You don't have to exert yourself. The only thing you need to do the first week is simply go to school.

Note that I did not say to attend class, be attentive, read or ask questions, and complete homework.

Also, I didn't tell you to that you go to the gym and workout, nor did I even suggest that you go to the gym, and work up the sweat... The only thing I told you was to visit the gym and take off. The process could take anywhere from 5 to 60 minutes.

Since this technique is simple and easy to follow it will make your brain not be able to fight back with the same intensity ... The emphasis should be on "fight your opponent as hard."

Over time, you'll be familiar with being there and then you can start to see outcomes.

Why?

Let's suppose that the muscles are sore from doing exercises... and your brain is trying to keep the exercise. It's likely that you regularly go to the gym on a regular basis. If you go at the gym exhausted and exhausted, your personal trainers from GOLD's GYM say there's a 99.8 percentage chance you'll work up a sweat.

The soreness eventually will fade as you become an exercise addict.

Chapter 16: Eternal Health

I think that everyone has the skills to achieve success.

When you read to now I'm sure you've said to yourself:

"Duh this is common sense."

"I already have all this information."

"He's not saying anything but"the obvious."

In a way I think you're correct.

In conclusion, I think that every person already knows how to be successful.

The purpose of the book's goal isn't just to teach the reader new things. It's about encouraging you to act on what that you already know.

Many people have been from seminar to seminar or bought several books, written notes in pages, and spent hours watching videos, and yet haven't reached the success that they had been told they would achieve.

The world of today is one where we are able to access all the data that we'd ever need. The information we need on any subject is one Google search, Wikipedia or a YouTube videos just a click away.

In the present, you can discover books, podcasts or websites. There are also seminars and workshops about how you can become millionaire, find an ex-girlfriend, buy six packs...

There's an abundance of broken individuals today. Why don't they go to the bookstores and purchasing the books they want and become financially self-sufficient?

America is now the world's most obese nation. the world. What is the reason why aren't all overweight individuals exercising? Aren't they aware that they need to exercise?

I'm sure you've gotten the idea...

All of us have all necessary information to make whatever decision they wish to accomplish in their lives.

In the event that you inquire of 10 persons this moment if they're aware of the fact that a healthy diet and regular exercise can make them healthier They'll all say yes. Ask them if they are actually eating healthy food and going to the fitness center? It's likely that 7/10 of them will are not going to answer and offer an "good justification" for why they don't.

I think everyone is aware of how to be successful, but I'm not convinced that they possess the capacity to use and apply the skills they've acquired.

"Knowing isn't enough, we have to apply."

Bruce Lee

"There's the difference between knowing the right path and actually walking it."

Morpheus

This is what the book is all about...

The question I like to get people to answer is what are two options to ensure that a person is physically fit?

The child might say, "Eat my vegetables and go outside to play."

You'd be right.

The only way to stay physically fit is through adequate nutrition and exercises.

Sure, you could refer to other aspects however, ultimately all of it can be considered a mere substitute or artificial form of healthy nutrition and exercise.

It is true that certain diseases have a genetic cause... I have a baby sister had sickle cells anemia when she was born as well as the medications she has to take ... Doctors still advise drinking plenty of water and fruit as well as a balanced diet.

What ever disease or condition that you suffer from or illness you've brought on yourself, exercising and eating right could help you get rid of it, or at times, reduce it so as to make it virtually irrelevant to your daily life.

Take a moment to think about this...

What number of depressed individuals have you encountered who exercise and eat a healthy diet daily?

While some can be very effective at exercising frequently, a lot of people cannot be able to keep a balanced diet also.

In order to eat well to be healthy, there is no need for a trendy diet. We do not require any supplements, and we don't require anything special for space or military food products.

The only thing we have to accomplish all we have to do ...

Surprise, surprise!

Use the exact system you just learned about:

1. Our mindset should support our objective

2. Show yourself

Contrary to exercising, in which you can easily see the many benefits that go along with it, there's specific skills and behaviors which require a deeper knowledge of how they will help you or keep your back from achieving it if you do not implement it into your daily day-to-day life.

A little greater understanding in order to be more conscious of the dangers.

The first level of awareness

The majority of food that consumed is a poison. This is a quote from Darren Hardy, author of the compound effect, editor of the magazine Success, as well as a world-renowned success coach. A majority of food available nowadays is a product of processing and manufacturing BS. Indeed, the proposition 65 of California stipulates that all food shops and retailers must identify every food item that could cause cancer. It's awe-inspiring to realize that a lot of people are dependent on their autopilots that they do not ever bother to learn about the possibility that chips they buy could cause cancer. Many of you are thinking to yourself "oh, you're right. I've eaten hot Cheetos for years and I'm good." But, you should recognize that you've gotten into an eating habit that involves eating cancer-causing chips but the most frightening part is that it's likely you're having other meals that could trigger cancer, too! You could consume 5-10 snacks a week which may lead to the development of cancer... However, I'm certain you'll be safe because nothing negative occurs to you ever? ?

I'm not trying in any way to off you, but I'm just trying to get you awake.

Darren Hardy says to go into your kitchen and get out the chips, cookies, or anything else and then read the nutritional information in the rear. It will include things like Niacin, riboflavin, the high-fructose corn syrup...

Hardy recommends that if you do not know the meaning of something and you don't know what it is, toss it out since it's a poisonous.

It may seem drastic, but the reality is that drastic times require drastic measures.

It is a matter of how serious are you about your well-being?

Are you looking forward to having the energy to spend more time with your kids, be affectionate to your spouse, and be more focused on your job?

Do you want to never be ever again sick? Would you like not having to travel to a miserable hospital, sit for long hours in a waiting room full of negative and sick people and then be treated by a doctor who doesn't make time to take the time to give you the care you deserve? which means you're left with a bag full of medication or a bandage on the I.V. which is to help you rehydrate in the bag, and within is a note saying:

Rest well Good nutrition, rest, as well as exercise! ?

Once you've eliminated everything which is harmful to your health or contains ingredients aren't clear to you and you've raised your consciousness. This means that when you go to the grocery store again and purchase food... You are aware that you're buying unhealthy foods. Now you're choosing to buy food items that cause cancer for your children. The simple realization of this will lead you to avoid buying harmful food items in the first instance.

With no bad food in the vicinity the area, you'll have a more chance of avoiding it.

In addition, habits are simpler to develop with the right percentages to our advantage.

First, you need to know is that food can be poisonous. Eliminate it. You'll be one step closer to being healthier because bad foods is gone.

A second awareness level for eating healthy

Set the expectation that your goals will never succeed unless you eat nutritious.

We'll say you'd prefer to become a doctor. From the time when you were little as a child, you've played the role of a nurse for your pet animals. In the grade level, you were awed studying anatomy as well as biology. One summer, your friend nearly drowned in an aquatic pool. He was saved from drowning by an EMT who had a good understanding of CPR Thanks to that medical professional, your most beloved friend is now alive. From that point on the only thing you've ever thought about was going to UCLA and study medicine. This is your love and your goal, it's the calling you have.

Let's imagine that I'm director of the UCLA medical school. I shoot a gun at your desire and inform you that in the event that you do not begin eating a healthy diet, I'll pull the trigger.

Imagine sitting at my desk and I'm telling you, listen Carla I know you have good scores, excellent advice, but let me tell you the truth... Every one of the UCLA doctors consume healthy food everyday, and we at UCLA make sure that our doctors are held to the very highest standards. We are looking for the most and most focused, disciplined and caring people that truly want to make a an impact in the world who are working alongside us. If you're unable to be healthy, maybe it's not for the right person for you ... What's the reason you wouldn't you consider applying to USC? You'll find it easier there?

Imagine!

I've just informed you that everyone that does what you would like to do is like this If you're not inclined to follow that path and kick the rocks!

How determined, motivated are you? How focused and persistent are you about eating healthily right now?

Red Pill:

Arnold Schwarzenegger, one of the few men living in this day and age who achieved everything he's desired... bodybuilding champion, highest-paid Hollywood celebrity Real estate mogul governor of the best state in the Union and was even was married to Kennedy. Kennedy states,

"Whatever it takes, I'll take on."

It should be the mindset you adopt!

Chapter 17: The Secret To Eating Healthy

It's not the difficult task as some think it is. It's just a bit harder than doing your workout since you're dealing many different things to consider.

Make an effort to grasp what I am saying...

The author of the book Born Rich, Bob proctor declares that success is an edge.

The distinction between places 1 and 2 could be just 1 second. Losing and winning could boil all down to an inch, one step of extra effort, a small amount of work.

Similar to this, the concept has a strong correlation with being healthy and eating well.

Many times, when people attempt to eat healthier often, they will make some extreme changes to their eating habits... There are bizarre modern-day things such as a no fruits and carbs or a diet with only 2000 calories Paleo, Atkins...

The whole thing is unneeded and, I believe, will not be effective for very the long. In the end, you'll be sabotaging your self for two weeks you reward yourself with the chance to cheat. This cheat day eventually transforms into a week the next month, the next thing you know, you're back at McDonald's.

NOTE: Never take a break or cheat during the first 2 months of making a habits.

Why?

Since the old habits are being used. Thus, a cheat day really is reinforcing the old habits.

Steps to take in order for a healthy diet is to:

Surprise, surprise!

"Just be sure to show up."

We're not planning to make many radical changes in our eating habits, but we'll make "razors edge" changes to our diet.

We can begin by creating an habit of drinking water more often.

The only thing we need to learn to accept drinking only water when we are at the same place, or at a specific meal.

Example 1.

I love learning in Starbucks each and each time I visit Starbucks I request a water. It's literally every time. Then I make a request for water without considering the idea.

Example 2.

Choose a meal at which there is no water consumed during the entire food. For breakfast, let's take it. Therefore, for the next month drinking water only to eat breakfast. In the next month, you can try the same breakfast and lunch. after which you can you can add dinner.

If taking a direct route to the water is not feasible, try a different route. Other methods may be employed. There is no correct or incorrect approach to " simply appear". It could mean different things for different individuals.

Don't forget, simply being there is not the most simple thing you can do. What could you do to make this is easy for you?

The suggestions I've given are just a few ideas of ideas that could be implemented.

With regards to the food we eat, things are more simple.

In the end, we'll only apply the razors edge.

Most people love potato chips. It was interesting to come to bean chips in a grocery store. I perused the label and after altering the vegetable chip, the new ones were rich in fiber as well as protein. The flavor was also amazing and almost tasted like the tortilla chip...

Are you a fan of fried chicken? Have a grilled chicken

You like fries? Eat sweet potato fries

Are you a fan of white rice? Brown rice is a good choice.

Are you a fan of peanuts? Eat trail mix

You like candy bars? Consume energy bars

You like candy? Eat dried fruit, energy fruit snacks, or workout fruit snacks

By making just a tiny change you could significantly alter the results.

"Yeah But justice eating well is pricey."

Well, that's fine, but who does the cost of medical care...

You can either pay for health insurance or

Or

Choose healthier foods that will boost your energy levels as well as happiness levels and your general well-being.

in Tom Corley's "Change your Habits, Change your Life," he said that the DNA of your body alters as you begin developing new habits throughout your daily life. When it comes to eating healthily Your taste buds adapt to the foods that you're consuming.

One of my friends told me that after having sandwiches in place of hamburgers for several days... "I attempted to re-visit and eat the burger but it didn't taste great, so I was about to vomit from the taste."

It's amazing that your body's physiology can alter to the point that it will reject food that is BS foods. However your body's chemistry can shift to the point that you begin to appreciate salads, fruit, water as well as grilled meat.

Red pill:

It is simple to eat healthy when you look at it from an appropriate view.

We're not asking that you make drastic modifications to your eating habits.

Make sure to make the changes that razor's edge.

Anything you consider to be the most simple thing you can do.

You can do this for approximately one month, then shift bit more.

The idea of drinking juice rather than soda is a fantastic way to do it...

Perhaps you begin with Tampico but then move on into Welch's and then Simply Orange 100 percent juice.

What's cool about this is that your taste buds will begin to help reinforce the new habit that you have made.

Your body's attempt to make you do exactly the same thing, by trying to make you appreciate the flavor of your actions.

Why?

Since your brain wants to be energy efficient by having auto-response to certain things.

We now know that, we can apply this knowledge to benefit ourselves.

Welcome!

The chapter also has a bonus section that you can read on the next page...

Imagine it as a an incentive to thank you thanks for taking the time to read this.

Chapter 18: Why Theory?

The term "theory" refers to a collection of theories and speculations which are derived from the study of natural phenomena. It attempts to understand the cause of the phenomena as well as their potential future behavior. In order to prove the validity of a theory you must follow the different steps of the scientific process.

But, we create speculations constantly. time everyday when we observe our mom walking into the front door with a rage It is an attempt in order to understand what caused her anger and what she's likely to do over the coming minutes. When you observe something, look into the reason what caused it.

WHY SOCIOLOGICAL?

It aims to understand and predict human behavior and preferences, specifically through focusing on the aspects of gender selection as well as power relationships between male and female.

A distinction needs to be drawn: one is a formal or logical theory while the other is a sociological one, as they're fundamentally different concepts. The term "formal theory" is known as a "scientific" theory like Einstein's theory of relativity. It attempts to clarify gravity, the motion of light, and the movement of celestial objects. Theories of formality are organized with a logic and rigid method, for example math, physics or chemistry, also known as "hard sciences.".

One of the most crucial things to be aware of is that a theory of science accepts no exceptions. In the event that there's an observation or experiment which proves the contrary that theory, it is incorrect or, to be better put, disproved (Popper's rule of falsifiability). Let's look at the instance of gravity. We know that if are holding a pen hands and open our fingers, the pen will fall onto the ground, since theories of relativity claims that objects draw each other by their weight. If at any point, you let go of the pen and it flies upwards, flying about, then the theory of relativity is not true which means we're back at the beginning, which means it is necessary to come up with another theory to explain how the pen can fly.

Let's look at another scenario within the engineering field. If a structure is that was constructed with the "Hello" method and then out of the clear blue, it comes down and without any catastrophe or earthquake in any way, this is a sign that other structures constructed using this same method are risky. The structure that has collapsed as an exception and a reason to be concerned about.

Sociological theories however is a study of human behavior and how we, as humans, may be different, and take different actions, such as market options, choices in life, for instance.

WHY STATISTICS?

Since red pill isn't founded on scientific or physical evidence from which we can draw thematic and empirical evidence instead, it is based on the human behavior and the way that people behave, with exceptions being commonplace. Therefore, it is necessary to determine the proportion of people who behave the way we expect as well as how many not and then draw statistics.

It's the same with medicine. Imagine 100 people suffering from headaches. Everyone takes an anti-histamine then the following day 90% of them are healthy and 10 do not. If 10 people are still suffering from headaches doesn't suggest that the medication is not effective, but it isn't a proof that is in contradiction to the theories. This means the medication works at 90. It is not the case that this exception does make any sense, and in fact should be anticipated.

It is the distinction between generalizing and absolutizing. Absolutizing is saying that all women love men with money'. It is not difficult to debunk this claim It is all you need to look for a woman that does not care about cash. In contrast saying that women are like men who have money is a broad statement that is a attempt to explain a universal behavior that is performed by a huge number of people, or a trend'. A single instance isn't enough. To counter this assertion, you must demonstrate that the vast majority of women aren't looking for men who are wealthy as I perceive it difficult, especially considering how the rich old guys get flooded by gold miners.

Stereotypes are nothing but social theories of generalisation. which means that you notice an action and then describe the behavior. However, this does not mean this is a true stereotype however, to use an exception that is based on the traditional one to disprove the notion is naive and useless. Let's take a case of a popular image: Americans are fat and are prone to eating poorly. Do you believe this? It is true, as per the CDC (a US public health institution) the rate of obesity among US residents is 42%. Who can say how many of them are "only obese. The generalisation is confirmed by the statistical analysis of the entire population. This does not mean the case that if I tell you "ah you can see the thin American" and everyone Americans seem to suddenly be skinny.

Can it be said that the red pill is a science? At best the red pill cannot be considered to be a "hard science'.

Is the red pill believed to be an objective test? It is not true that the theory behind it can be considered to be objective (it is not difficult to find research studies in the academic world that demonstrate the effects of beauty on attraction) However, the explanations for the reasons and why are contested and are difficult to prove.

Is it possible to say that the red pill is scientific? It is, but it's difficult to understand, somewhat similar to psychology. Both are founded on objectively observable information (e.g. that loss of employment causes anxiety, or that loss of a loved one can trigger mood swings, and other scenarios) However, in order to clarify the reasons behind why people behave in this an approach or even the best way to help those suffering from certain illnesses Good luck in proving this as unbiased.

Chapter 19: Why Descriptive?

Red pill is a description of it, and only provides bare details, and that's all it is. It's the end. There is no reference to political, or even social goals. Nor does it specify the way to behave.

This is what really irritates me. I've always been astonished by the absurdity of "Oh red pill is seeking to go back to the patriarchy'. It's impossible to find anything more false.

The red pill is a source of details about the way people have a sexual attraction and how they conduct themselves. When you think 'it did better in the days of patriarchy' then it's the individual conclusion, and one's personal company.

Consider the Bible as well as the Catholic faith as an illustration since at the end of the day, it is a sociological concept. There's a philosophical base (God made the universe in just seven days, and created humans are created in their basic and recognizable form as well as.) In addition, there's an ethical code (the Ten Commandments, the model of Jesus) and then there are goals for the earth (evangelising people and drawing individuals closer to the Church) as well as otherworldly goals (i.e. that of the rewards in paradise). Red pill does not have code of conduct and neither do they have political or social goals and even spiritual purposes. This is simply information, possibly right or wrong however nothing else. It has been reported that it is believed that the red pill is a cult and that the people must be free to act according to their own preferences. However, who can tell you any of this? You can do what you want to.

An example that is practical, The LMS theory is that a woman selects men who have the best potential LMS. The theory suggests a range of options to choose from: you can reach the maximum L through surgery or training and then devote greater time and effort to earn more income. You may decide that there is no value or accept that he's unattractive to females and turn into a MGTOW. Another may claim to be rich with a certain type of cash and be sexually attractive despite having a financial debt. Another one may decide that the cash will spend it on prostitutes rather than investing it in nice clothing and impressing the puella pulcra in the midst of duty. It's their choice. Personal choice and effects, after they have learned the details of a particular piece is the responsibility of the person who made the decision.

All of this puts an end to the false notion of a resemblance between redpilled and incel.

Being red pilled is the irrational assumption of one who has a knowledge of red pills and claims to be one active and voluntarily.

Incel is, on the other hand is an existential, passive condition experienced by people because of being a person with the lowest LMS or a sexy personality and a social environment where the demands of women are excessive, resulting in being out from the world of sexual relations.

WHY PROBABILISTIC?

The most frequent mistake made by those who have recently read about the LMS theory is to believe "oh well, then people who are ugly aren't laid-back, but gorgeous folks do'. It's not true the red pill doesn't make decisions based on absolutes, rather, it is based on probabilities: it doesn't state that if someone is attractive, you are likely to get laid. But it is true that the prettier someone is, the greater his chance of getting laid. There certain men with ugly faces who tend to be more likely to get laid than beautiful men, however, they're not many in. Similar to the female sexual power. If women are your thing, then is more likely to possess more sexual strength than men however, it's not necessarily the case. Always think using probabilities.

A completely random scenario with driving It's not like when one drives when driving at a speed that is over speeds, then immediately traffic police are on the scene and penalize the driver. However, the faster one goes and the more likely it is of getting caught.

The market for sexual services is survival and reproduction.

A metaphor that I prefer to employ to describe the interactions between males and women is the market for sexual relations.

Sexual relations between males and females can be described metaphorically as a huge market where women and men trade their reproductive and sexual value with the goal of building the possibility of a short-term or long-term partnership that could benefit both parties.

As you would when you are planning to buy a new car, and you realize that you'll need select one that's less expensive than the amount you've got at the bank, when you look for a lady, you'll need to consider the value of your sexuality and have the money to buy an individual who's worth significantly more than the amount you afford to offer.

The value of sexual market is what gives you the ability to influence on other people and control the actions of others. This power is known as Sexual Power.

But, it must be made clear that the sexual market value isn't the same as the value of a human being. It's not something which is paid to a individual, but instead the person's prospective beauty.

There are two distinct aspects to consider. Although we often place our self-esteem in relation to our appearance and how attractive we are, I'd like to emphasize that, on this site, both aspects are considered entirely separately, which means that there could be beautiful people with an extremely low value on the market and slender individuals who look stunning.

The logic behind attraction is distinct from the principles which determine the human characteristics.

Once we have established this, let's go and find out what value will be based upon.

Women's market value is in large part influenced by fertility and beauty, the value of a man's product is mostly based on the appearance and social status of his family, the triad of familiarity that creates LMS theory. LMS theory.

The reason for these characteristics is the notion that a human's existence is defined by two primary objectives: Reproduction and Survival.

Beauty and fertility affect the value of reproduction, i.e. having the capacity to provide healthy genes to children, and thus develop well-nourished and robust, while both status and money are tied to the value of survival, as the rich person, who has greater resources, is less likely to drink early.

If you've noticed that men make their choices about sexuality mostly on women's reproductive potential, while females tend to base their choices depend on survival as well as reproductive worth.

That means that someone who's appearance isn't the best is able to make up for it for it with status and money but still look at ease (this should be the case at least but in actual practice, it's quite complicated) however, men tend to put less emphasis on women's status.

Between a wealthy 5 and a poor 7, males will most likely towards the former, but the option between a wealthy 5 and a poor seven isn't so clear.

What is crucial, however to remember is that the choices we make to support other people or avoid them from them, be it in an intimate or romantic relation, is influenced by the possibility of enhancing or reducing our capacity to live and reproduce.

Chapter 20: Demand And Supply

Just like any other market in general, the market of sexual relations is also affected by demand and supply. When it comes to sexual interactions, the supply and demand is governed by polygamy as well as hypergamy.

There's an enormous need for females (polygamy) and polygamy, in the context of a very restricted supply of men that have higher price (hypergamy).

The female is in the supply-side and has a greater average market value than a man that creates an disparity between males and females in addition to between men with higher value and less valuable males.

This is a consequence of the notorious'sexual freedom which is a dream of feminists. It has led couples to an absolute chaos where some males (around 20% in my estimates) enjoy the favors of a majority of women, while the remaining women fight over who gets the favours which is the exact opposite of what was the case in past days when marriage and family was an equalizer for society.

After the decline of the importance of marriage, and the potential of sexual relations that were not committed high-value males were more inclined to engage in less-value women, effectively diminishing their opportunities and raising the worth of women.

Men who remain have been remaining with just three options to follow:

1.Take your crumbs from marketplace, i.e. some of the most sexiest ladies, despite possessing perhaps the average LMS

2.Retire from the marketplace and focusing on other hobbies

3.Turning towards an alternative market i.e. prostitution.

The reality is that those who don't have LMS standards to find the girls of their choice are required to pay for them.

But, in reality it's not true to state that he "pays the fucks, as there can be no such thing as an unpaid fool. Everybody pays, not just those who are beautiful. However, they make use of a distinct type of currency, one that is aesthetics.

The beauty industry is something that is a product like money and for everything else a monetary asset but our society believes it is a crime to get a woman hiring her to gain money-making opportunity, whereas it is a source of credit for the women who are attractive being lucky enough to get their bones on the proper location.

From this point where I would suggest we restart our efforts to restore fairness in this market we have described in our article: begin by making prostitutes socially acceptable as well as affordable for males.

Get over the hurdle of feminists who have generally opposed prostituting because of the convenience. Their interest in protecting themselves from exploitation is minor compared to being able to see their value reduce because of prostitution's competition.

The possibility of being capable of using prostitutes at a low cost quickly, without hassle and with no any stigmatisation from society, those with higher worth are not enticed to sell out. A greater equilibrium in sexual relations would be brought back.

The whole thing without jeopardizing women's rights to make their own choices by limiting her choices to reasonable demands.

Hypergamy and Polygamy They are what they sound like and how do they affect your sexual life

What are the main differences between women and men? How does the female brain work? The same for men.

Imagine that 10 men and 10 women with the same appearance degree are on an island in the desert, wrecked as Robinson Crusoe and without chance of recovering in any time very soon. They've got a long time before them, during which they must survive and coordinate their activities through collaboration.

However, they're still humans and are, therefore, guided by a certain set of impulses.

What happens during such an event? What would be the difference between them? What will be the group dynamics that change? Following the initial period of settling in where the group settles down and divide the assignments according to the individual's abilities and strengths, specific physical needs will start to be felt. And slowly, relationships of love and sexuality between women and men are likely to develop. This is where the character of both comes into play the polygamous male and hypergamous in women.

Contrary to popular belief are not performing the same sort of sexual choice.

It is due to the fact that the two species are genetically different and play different roles.

The female is in charge of procreation, while the male is in charge has the responsibility of conceiving.

Based on everything, it's evident that it is essential that a man try to get more women pregnant in order to reach the goal. A woman, who has the potential of having a baby, and capable of being fertilized by just one person is not interested in having a relationship with anyone, but to men who have a greater rate of survival and a higher value for reproduction. (Parental Investment Theory, Trivers 1972].

The tendency of men to look for a variety of females is known as polygamy. Women's tendencies to be extremely specific, especially within the red pillsphere is known as hypergamy.

It is clear that these tendencies fall from a culture and social pressure to fight them, but it isn't of importance to us as we're looking at an environment as it exists as it is in its original state.

What will this mean for the island? This will mean that around,

Two men from these 10 (the most attractive, the toughest hunter) are the top 8 females (see Pareto principle)

The two women who remain can get a little lost with the 5-6 other males in the group (always in search of the highest two)

The remaining males will be totally cut off from the possibility of any romantic relationship.

In this instance, I think, what is it that could inspire these men (the marginalized) to join forces for their group's interests? Put yourself into the shoes of one of them. They do your best throughout the day, hunt and capture a rabbit but with a lot of difficulties (it is known as the infamous island where vegans argue) and at night, you must to pass it on to other members of the group. You may even share it those women who reject the idea.

Who is the one who makes you do it?

Humanity isn't your energy, and you're being the victim and your genes will be destined for the end of time, and it could even be every person to himself, and everyone else stick.

There could be worse scenarios and the outcasts could have a desire to dominate the other contestants, as one male from the middle class could be keen on taking two of the best to be able to join the top.

We are not living in an ideal society where there aren't any rules, policemen or judges. Just nature's laws like in the animal kingdom. The situation could be extremely challenging, more so because there is an evident disparity in privileges for both genders as, in such a situation, males will be required perform all the heavy labor, like shifting stones, constructing houses and hunting, whereas women can do routine tasks like collecting fruit or getting water.

What happens now?

The result is that one among the men of the group, perhaps one among the most intelligent thinks of a smart concept and decides to divide women equally between the men. Every man is allowed to only have one female, and the reverse is true.

Although this may appear at first glance, but there is no guarantee that the two most stylish men are going to continue to have a romantic relationship with their female counterparts However, of course this time they're doing so at the risk of their own lives because a structure of society is in place to blame the behavior of these two men.

All males in the island feel energized to get their work done, and the tiny group grows and enjoys better life conditions and advances in technology that are beneficial to all. In this case, it's the summing up of the birth of patriarchy one of the institutions that has been so widely blamed yet was vital to attain the standards of living that we today enjoy.Let us take a trip back to our home island and imagine that instead of surviving in poverty, survivors of the shipwreck have a comfortable life, because at the time of the wreck, plenty of meals and other necessities are also ashore.

The labor of attractive males would not be required and the social system could be established in which women are in the lead in the society, as for as long as there are resources available.

In the present, Western society is facing the second possibility, that it is currently consuming everything it had accumulated previously and, in large part, Western men have become socially useless'. This provides fertile ground for feminist movements of all kinds and movements, which are the only consequence of the economic prosperity of our times and will not be seen to expand even in the midst of hard times.

However, the resources do not come in endless quantities, as the increasing number of people who subscribe to a patriarchal conception of social life arrive to us, and demanding their resources (after all the majority of us Westerners who are softer because of affluence are not parents anymore) and contributing to the exhaustion of their resources.

After all of it has been done, in a couple of years, the period of bliss for women sexual experience will be one of those memories. Then we'll be back to our earlier state and the man who was deemed inferior will be able to regain his worth.

Chapter 21: The Pitcairn Experiment

It's the month of January and a small group of English sailors arrived on the beaches of an isolated, uninhabited island situated in the Pacific Ocean.

It is the time of exploration, however the leader Fletcher Christian is no ordinary explorator, and what's more than the vessel that carried him there named the Bounty and its crew just a few months before was the reason for one of the most famous mutinies that has ever occurred in the time of the British navy. However, let's go further back in time.

The Bounty was sailed from the shores of England on December 17, 1787 under the command of Captain William Bligh. The mission is to sail towards Tahiti, the Polynesian Island of Tahiti for the purpose of acquiring seeds from a native plant known as the "breadfruit tree" and the fruit is set to provide a cheap source of income for slaves in the British colonies of Central America.

The life of the crew is quite difficult, not in the least due to Bligh is deciding to go to take the shortest route i.e. heading west, and then endeavor to get around Cape Horn.

It's a risky venture, which has a low chance of success. It engulfs the Bounty within the turbulent currents to the to the south from Tierra del Fuego for a satisfactory month. However, captain decides to abandon ship and tells the crew to return to the Cape of Good Hope.

The British arrived in Tahiti in the month of October 1788, and instantly received a friendly welcome.

The crowd was a festive one of the locals who eagerly greeted the latest visitors to

Matavai Bay and a party was held in the evening that included dance and music in honor of guests.

They are shocked to learn they're required to remain there for months at a time which is because that's the time is needed for the fruit's ripening in this time the guys go crazy particularly with local ladies.

In the Tahitian society that prevailed at the time the women are allowed total freedom to sexually engage, while men frequently exchange wives, and refusing to share intimate moments with them can be thought to be insensitive. In fact, even the British were able to benefit from this practice that was completely contrary to the customs they were accustomed to back in their homeland.

Every seaman has at the very the very least one female companion who entertains him. The officers have more simultaneously. time.

Based on the travel stories it is clear that there's a hedonistic scene which is a very relaxed and sane life full of orgies and activities.

Whites are regarded as appealing due to their beautiful skin tone, regardless of their facial characteristics.

Certain, like the Captain Samuel Wallis who came to the island a mere twenty years prior were even victimized by erotic harassment from local women.

These are outlined by the Captain James Cook in the following sentences:

"The women from the upper class are larger than our normal, while those from lower class are shorter than we. Women of the highest rank their complexions are dark, the skin is smooth and smooth and soft. Faces are beautifully shaped and is often stunning, eyes that are expressive and glowing, but now it appears to melt in sweet. The teeth are regular and clear with no unpleasant breath smooth and relaxed movements. They're exceptionally well-maintained: they clean them from head to foot every day three times, beneath the numerous

There are waterfalls in the island as well as at mealtimes they clean their hands and mouths. Their smiles are never rough and never tainted by fear and their behavior is amiable and welcoming. They act with the confidence of people who don't think that they need to remain vigilant against anybody or anything.

Kind to each other as well as when it comes to strangers, gentle and gentle, they don't get offended and don't have anger issues. Hands and arms are delicately formed even though they are without shoes, they have feet that aren't rough or unshapely'.Paul GauguinWhere are we from? What are we? What are we doing? (1897)

On that island located on the opposite part of the globe those modest English volunteer who were there to make a few dollars and discovered paradise. So it is not surprising that in the years to come, numerous Europeans were drawn to Tahiti only to become affected by the "Tahiti illness'. The artist Paul Gauguin, who almost one century later made his way towards the Polynesian archipelago in order to make the location the backdrop for his artwork, however he was somewhat dismayed to discover that the island was now changed into Frenchified and the customs of its past were almost gone.

The Mutiny of the Bounty

After having spent a few months in such a beautiful environment, eating exotic fruits and fish with ladies who are treated with the respect of queens, it's easy to envision the thought of being forced to go back to the solitary existence of humble biscuits and relentless work according to the orders from a possibly overly enthusiastic superior officer and going to an area where they were in the lowest rung of socially privileged, surely wasn't very attractive.

On the return journey, the crew members appear anxious and, at some moment the tension gets so strong that the officer Christian revolts against Captain along with the other crew members joins in a rebellion.

The consequences of this decision are grave, because for mutineers, there's death penalties through hanging. The step was taken now and the captain is left in the sea in a tiny lifeboat having only his sextant, and some supplies.

In spite of all odds and his youth, likely driven by a deep desire to retaliate, Bligh can survive going on a two-month voyage in the absence of food in hundreds of miles of water lined with islands home to cannibals. He then reaches Timor, the Dutch colony in Timor and writing about what's transpired.

The mutineers are back in Tahiti and unloaded certain men who were committed to Bligh however were unable to board the lifeboat that was overfilled.

However, they know that Tahiti is where they'd look for them. So they take their female companions along with the other Polynesian males onboard and set out for a safe place to call home.

The quest is long and never ends: the islands they encounter on their travels are often inhospitable and not having enough vegetation or water. Other times, they are filled with hostile people.

The search for answers is futile as they eventually discover an island that isn't shown on maps.

Actually, it's an island that has been discovered, Pitcairn. In the official maps of the British navy it is located, but its position is marked by 160-mile errors and this means they will only find the island by accident. This is the ideal location to avoid English law, not to mention due to the fact that

Pitcairn isn't just uninhabited and is also rich in fruits, game as well as fresh water sources and also has a coastline that is not able to allow vessels to dock.

The British escapees and their comrades arrive and burn the Bounty to block it from being spotted by the British navy from spotting the vessel. It's the start of a new chapter in their lives.

The colonists number 28 total. Fiveteen males (nine English and six natives) and 12 women and a little girl. However, coexistence isn't always an easy task. How do you ensure social order is preserved in a small group located on an isolated island with no authority to make sure that laws have been observed?

What follows is fascinating from an anthropological point perspective. More men are there than women, and the British divide the women, while treating the

Polynesians, who later some time, rebel to be treated as slaves.

Within three years due to the constant competition among the males, many members of the crew already murdered each other as a kind of aggressive self-regulating mechanism that was that was triggered by the social tension which had been created.

When the Polynesians have been exterminated and gone, one of the last survivors dubbed John Adams, evidently the most popular of the entire group, discovers an avenue to find a way of reconciling with the men who are left and bring peace back to the island time. After the demise of the last mutineers Adams remains the sole man living on the island. He manages the tiny community comprised of just ten women and 23 youngsters influenced by the tenets of the religion. He teaches residents with the help of texts from the Bounty.

In 1814, an British navy vessel rediscovered Pitcairn around 1814 everybody across the UK was so amazed by this outlaw's retribution and ability to establish and lead a modest but economically prosperous group of citizens peacefully living together, they accepted his sins and gave the island the status of a stately colony. Today, Pitcairn is inhabited by people who were the descendants of mutineers from the Bounty and is a living testament to the reality of Fletcher Christian and his companions their dream of freedom.

Consider imagining a situation with two isolated islands at sea On one, there are just men. Let's suppose a random number of people of them, the typical average comprising people aged between 5-7. The other is women's version to this group i.e. 10 random females aged who are between the ages of 5 and 7. Both islands are separated, and they can't meet up when they visit one island, but they will be able to see what's going on at the other side of the island.

In this instance, we decide to place an 8-year-old woman on the island for men and a male of 8 on the female island. What will happen? What happens if:

The woman could make use of her sexual strength to have all males twirl for her. she'd be an emperor without a care in the world and would not give her self to one of the males while taking in the 8 in the opposite island and trying to connect with him due to some reason.

Men would be fighting for her attention and each would be trying to appear attractive in front of the other There would be some insecurity between them. They might even harm the other over time.

In the end, the woman who was finally conscious that she was not able to be the one to have it all, would choose to be the most shabby of group members and choose the woman who appeared more attractive and/or proved to be more adept at fishing or hunting and/or had more leadership capabilities in the group.

However on the opposite island, the gentleman was even willing to let women take care of him and honor him but they would be stamped by him beginning at the most gorgeous then ending with the ugly before, after getting bored of them the sexiness, he would begin to nag him about the insanity of being able to have the eight in the opposite island and constantly thinking about her.

This is the meaning of Hypergamy and Polygamy refer to.

Sexual power

"Nature has granted women so powerful power, that law has judiciously given them very little." -Samuel Johnson (1709-1784)

Today, I'm going to talk with you about one of the strongest factors that influence social relations: Sexual Power.

Sexual Power refers to the power which a person has to influence others and earn rewards through sexual appeal, i.e the value of his or her appearance in the marketplace of sexuality which is a common economic term employed in blogs to describe in general terms how social relations work and the way they occur by means of an exchange of value which could be the case between a buyer and seller on any market.

Sexuality is rooted in sexual relations, which gives an opportunity to have connections with a growing number of important sexual partner. But it is much beyond just the sexual side that it transversal, and allows for a higher standard of living in all aspects. This allows benefits to be enjoyed in the professional, economic social, and in general the entire realm of community living.

Sexual power is an evident concept, but it isn't yet officially accepted in our culture. When we describe the term "powerful" for a person the truth is that we're typically referring to their economic as well as social authority they possess.

Man is powerful because the position he is in lets him impose his will upon others or because he's got sufficient money to enjoy some privileges.

But, we don't think that someone has power just because they are attractive. and attractive.

Beauty represents the highest value an individual can enjoy within the realm of sexuality which is especially true for females while men as we've witnessed through this theory of LMS theory, continue to depend on status and money for a boost in their power sexually.

After introducing the notion of sexual power is now time to examine two aspects of the concept:

1.The acceptance of Sexual Power in our society

2.The Distribution of Sexual Power across sexes

While the sexual urge is the most intense which Mother Nature has given us and influences our decisions all the time however, there's an element of sexism in discussing it since a further division of society based on sexuality will result in an extreme gap and result in an array of inequalities that clearly don't fit the social way of life.

It is still a fact that discrimination happens at the in the end, but everybody is able to ignore it, and try to reduce the impact of it.

It is accepted as normal for bar owners, in hiring employees, to pick a gorgeous young woman who is able to draw patrons over an (possibly unattractive) boy even though they may both be superior when it comes to making cocktails.

You try to explain this, and then explain the person that such a decision is made based on the sexual capabilities of the employee who is to be hired and people are likely to consider that they were in awe.

Similar to the admission process and drinking in some bars. Contrary to many males, who get left out simply due to the fact that they don't have the right shirt, females often have free entry and pay no drinks. It is an obvious commercial decision because the greater number of women are there, the greater number of men will are enticed to attend the club.

This is an egregious discrimination and people don't stop to consider and invoke medieval notions like 'gallantry'.

Feminism is an expert in ignoring this issue and is leading the way in the discussion of male advantages (in the majority of cases, not even present) and attempting to portray women off as weak victim even though they're situated in an advantageous position.

Take the case of prostitution for example. Prostitution is typically described by feminists as the result of exploiting women's bodies. It's impossible to find a more untrue statement!

While ignoring the problem of the females who actually sexually exploited and who tend to be in the minority, the majority of prostitutes who engage in this type of business take advantage of their sexual strength.

They are the ones who swindle the males by taking advantage by the reality that an women on average have more sexual power because she's on the demand aspect of the sexual market. According to the old saying "a hairy blond in the direction of the uphill pulls much more than an entire ox cart on its descent'.

What are the number of women you know that are required to be paid for sexual gratification? Female customers are smaller, mostly older, dehydrated women that pay with the hotties of their youth and the male clientele's pleasure in prostitution spans all ages, including males of all ages, appearance, financial and social standing.

There is no reason why the prohibition of prostitution is fiercely opposed by feminists. Prostitution because it offers sexual sex for a price which is available at a greater or lesser cost to everybody and reduces women's power to sexually engage which obviously doesn't make a good impression on all feminist movements, which seem to be fighting to ensure equality but, in actuality they only care about conserving their own power and rights.

Consider what might be the consequences if one did be denied access to sexually oriented sex The result would cause chaos since the rivalry among men has already become embarrassing.

It is likely that rape will also grow however, feminists do not realize this.

Talking about rape, sexual violence is at the heart of feminism, and also one of the most important arguments that are used to demonstrate how women have a constant risk in the midst of a savage society constantly at the mercy of the male antagonist.

Afterward, attempt to take the same logic like the one you just heard regarding prostitution. Ask yourself the root of the violence committed by sexual assault. Yes, time, the more powerful female sexuality is the most powerful.

A higher likelihood of being raped one of the consequences of having more sexual strength.

It's a little similar to having money. If you're rich, you'll have the power to do more, however you are vulnerable to being a victim of being a victim of theft.

It is now a good idea to be able to access money, and then run the chance of having it taken from the person who has it (a chance that could be reduced if you employ some prudence and logic and stay clear of being at risk in particular situations) or to be poor, and run the risk, though less likely that of being targeted? The answer to this is pretty simple.

In this way, I'm not saying it's a good idea to take risks with the possibility of violence because you have the power of sexual or economic, I'm simply stating that it is how life is.

In the end, it's normal for women to not protest when her sexuality provides her with certain benefits and she slyly takes benefit of it and does not worry about the negative males' treatment.

Who is more powerful in sexuality in the relationship between women and men?

Determining who is the one with the highest sexual authority between males and females is an intricate issue that can't be dismissed as trivial. I'd suggest that in all likelihood, even with the same social and economic status women are more powerful in sexual strength, due to the fact that the women operate on the supply part of the equation.

To be able to manage sexual power, men must have money and Status, but an above average MS levels might not be sufficient. In the 20th year of their lives the your physical appearance matters more than status or social standing therefore, if we're speaking of men aged 20 and over, females are able to have a greater sexual influence over men.

In her 20s, a woman has an endless variety of choices as she is able to have fun even with guys who are better and attractive than her. A man in his 60s must put in an enormous amount of work however they will never be able to attain the same level as the men around him. It is only necessary to take a look at our study about sexual partners to realize that there is a huge difference in the sexual lives of a man in his 20s and woman. And in this case, I'd want to quote one of our users: Damned:

"We often discuss the disparities in income and social standing, etc. Many people believe it is false that there exist wealthy and extremely poor individuals. Therefore, the different redistributive practices of wealth. However, when we look at what is different between ugly and non-ugly on the subject of relationships to the other sex The majority (I refer to the most as I keep in mind that those who are people who are ugly, contrary to what people believe, is only a small percentage) are not just unable to consider it to be wrong, but aren't aware of that it is happening. However, these distinctions are more significant and unfair. It is more important due to the fact that I believe 99.99 percent of the population would prefer to have the hot lady at night as well as the Punto in the garage rather than the toilet at night (when it's not directly Federica the friendly hand) as well as the Ferrari inside the garage. Right? It's even more unfair since the beauty (of facial appearance) is a thing for which there is no error or merit. On the other hand, it is possible to earn money through dedication."

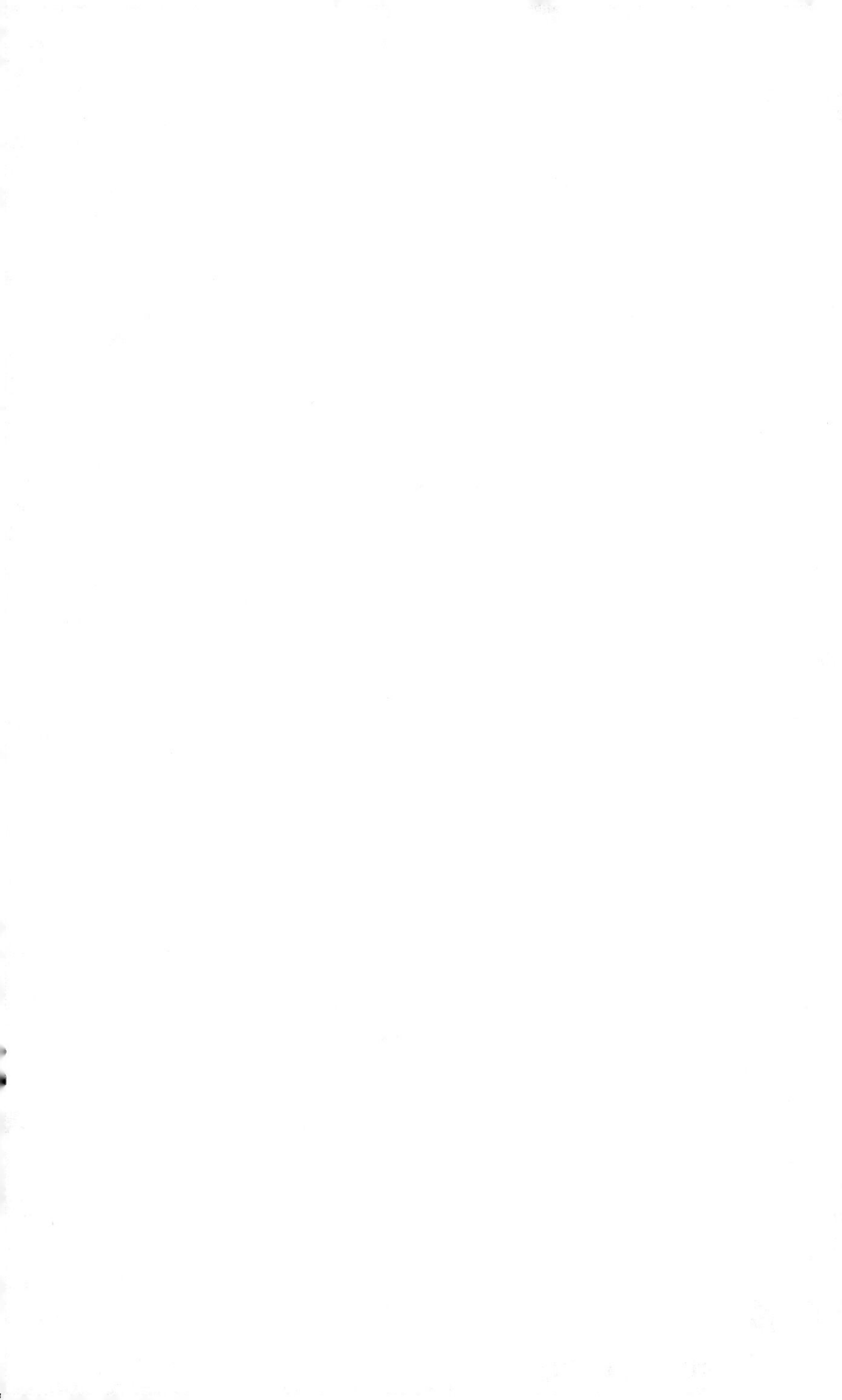